Physical Therapy
What PT Schools Are Not Teaching Their Students

By
Brian Grenda PT,DPT,CSCS,COMT

About The Author

My name is Brian Grenda and I am a licensed practicing physical therapist (PT), certified strength and conditioning specialist (CSCS), and certified manual therapist (COMT). I have been a physical therapist for over 5 years. I graduated from the University of Tampa in 2005 with a Bachelor's degree in exercise science and a minor in psychology. I attended NovaSoutheastern University (NSU) to obtain my doctorate of physical therapy (DPT). In 2009, I graduated from NSU and started working as a licensed PT in the state of Florida. I started working for Select Physical Therapy in the summer of 2009 and currently work for them now.

I will be the first one to admit that I am not the best physical therapist in the world or have all the answers when it comes to physical therapy. Through my experiences as a PT student, licensed staff physical therapist and center manager, I have developed simple effective ways to make your life as a therapist easier and increase the growth of your outpatient orthopedic PT business. I know when I was in PT school and started as a new graduate from PT school, I knew a lot of book material and school based knowledge about physical therapy but did not really know about the business of physical therapy and how a real world physical therapy clinic operates. That is why I wrote this book about how to be successful in PT and to teach people what PT schools are unfortunately not covering in their programs.

There are thousands of therapists in the U.S. and everyone can use a fresh perspective from a therapist about therapy from time to time. Hopefully some of these strategies, techniques, standards, and methods in this book are currently being performed by the majority of successful therapists. I feel that all therapists young and old can benefit from this book by following these simple strategies to help grow your business and treat patients safely, effectively, and efficiently.

I am not a college professor or guidance counselor but I do know what PT schools want in a potential student and require from their applicants. For any and all students who may need some guidance, help, or questions answered, your first stop should be your college advisor. Hopefully your college advisor is knowledge, available, and helpful. Unfortunately all advisors are not created equal and some may not be helpful at all. I luckily had a great Exercise Science advisor who helped me down the right path. I do not work for a University but want to be able to help students to become PTs or other medical professionals. You can find me on Facebook, Twitter @PTMadeSimple, and email at BrianG1221@hotmail.com. Feel free to contact me with questions, comments, or anything else. This book is intended to teach, educate, and provide an outlet for students and professionals to be the best PT that they can be. I have been successful in my young PT career and have found proven ways for everyone to be successful. Hope you enjoy this book and reach out to me with any questions, comments, or general communication. Thank you.

Content Chapters

Appendix

Chapter 1

Overview

This book was written to give a real world perspective of physical therapy from a physical therapist. The title is not meant to put down PT school but merely to catch the eye of potential PT students and anyone interested in physical therapy (PT) as a career. This book will be discussing what I feel are important areas of physical therapy that are barely taught in PT school or even omitted from the curriculum. This book will cover a lot of the material of how to be successful in outpatient orthopedics, including how to increase your outpatient orthopedic business and revenue, improve your evaluation and treatment skills, and educate about how to manage or work in a great work environment. This book is not intended to replace a PT degree or put down PT school but merely to educate about the flaws in the curriculum of PT school and what is not being taught to PT students. PT school is a necessary path to obtain a PT degree and to become a licensed therapist. PT school unfortunately does not cover any aspects of real world PT clinic situations and problems. PT schools do not teach someone how to treat two patients at once, how to find a job, how to manage your money while in PT school, or how to market and grow a PT business. This book is intended to be a great source of reference in addition to your PT school curriculum and education. This book will teach the real world PT material that is needed to be successful and not covered by PT schools.

This book unfortunately will not cover all areas of physical therapy, but will focus on important areas on how to be successful as a therapist. This book is intended to show how to become a successful staff therapist, physical therapy business owner, physical therapy student, and PT manager. We will be breaking down physical therapy into several different aspects that are necessary to be successful from a therapist treating patients stand point to the view of the patient and how a patient can reach their maximum rehab potential and enjoy coming to PT.

By following the easy concepts and strategies in this book, you will be able to grow as a PT student, business owner, practicing physical therapist, and/or center manager of an outpatient orthopedic clinic. Success is not guaranteed by any means but if you follow the proven steps in the book you will succeed in most if not all aspects of outpatient orthopedic physical therapy. Through our years of experience in the outpatient physical therapy setting we have come up with several easy proven concepts that any and all physical therapists from the new graduate to the seasoned veteran may benefit from.

After taking several students and practicing physical therapy for many years, I decided to write a book about physical therapy from a physical therapist perspective. I have been a student, a staff PT, and currently as a center manager of a clinic. Paying my dues and having many different experiences has shaped me into the therapist I am today. We thought people could benefit from the lessons we have experienced firsthand and learned from. I definitely do not want people to think that I have all the answers by any means but do want people to think about this book as a source to help them be a great successful physical therapist. Physical therapy is a very open ended career but certain things must be done to guarantee success with patients and the business of physical therapy. I believe we have a great method to manage both ends of the spectrum from the patient first PT to the business man who is driven by financial success and revenue. I feel that a great therapist should be a combination of both hands on patient driven success and the financial business person. As a center manager I need to be a mix of both in my clinic to be successful. I have worked hard, paid my dues, and found strategies that will help most clinics and patient populations.

So please enjoy the book and share the concepts and strategies with your fellow staff, students, and faculty. I am a firm believer that we have strength in numbers and if we follow the ideas of this book we can change the profession of PT for the better. Being a therapist is a great career and hopefully this book and ideas will make more people want to go into physical therapy and/or improve the profession. Thank you for taking the time for buying this book. Please refer others to purchase this book if you feel they might benefit from it.

Chapter 2

PT School

There are over 200+ PT schools in the continental U.S. currently and all of the programs are a doctorate of physical therapy (DPT). I graduated from physical therapy school in 2009 from one of the 10 PT schools in Florida with my doctorate in physical therapy and a good sense of physical therapy book knowledge. I knew the PT classroom material but did not really know the world of physical therapy from a clinical and business sense. As with most professions, physical therapy is a field that the more time and experience you put in the better you become. Physical therapy school is a 3 year program that is very stressful, educational, and fun but also very expensive.

PT school is a great time in your life and one last big hoorah before you hit the job market and real world. Most people go right from undergrad into grad school with a minimal summer break in between. Fortunately, I did not do that and was able to take a year off, move back home and save a year's income while living at home to save for PT school. I am glad that I had that opportunity because PT school is very expensive. I'm sure the cost per semester has increased since I went to school, but when I finished my 3 year long program, I owed around 100k in loans. That is with a part time job and saving money for about a year before going into PT school. My advice is to save money during undergrad and plan on spending about 100k plus living expenses, books, supplies, and miscellaneous items while in PT school.

For those who may not know, to get into a physical therapy school you first must complete a 4 year undergraduate degree and meet the requirements for acceptance. Most schools require a certain number of volunteer hours in physical therapy clinics, centers, or hospitals along with the prerequisite classes such as anatomy, biology, chemistry, and physics. My advice is to consult the school's website that you are interested in about their requirements and contact them with any questions. Every school will have a contact number and email, so you can reach them with any questions you might have.

Three years of education in the field of physical therapy will fly by. In PT school, you are always studying for some test, practical, project, or increasing your general knowledge. PT can be very stressful and challenging but that means you are growing and pushing yourself outside of your prior level of education and experience. PT school does a great job of having a mix of classroom material and hands-on experience based clinical internship learning. Some say you truly starting learning physical therapy when you enter the clinic during your clinical rotations and treat real patients. Classroom book material is the foundation of PT knowledge but putting it all together with real patients is priceless and how PT students truly learn how to be the best therapist that they can be.

Physical therapy school barely covers any aspects of the business side of PT. Students and new graduates from physical therapy school know very little if anything about the aspects of insurances, billing, and schedule productivity. I know why they don't cover it in PT school, but as an employer who will hire staff therapists it would benefit schools to teach their students a little bit more about the real world outpatient orthopedic business model. Hopefully all PT students will learn how to document properly, bill accordingly, and the business side of PT before they graduate. I know that I learned all of the Medicare guidelines, billing units, and insurance information during my clinical rotations. I am sure that is what PT schools rely on, but that is a big gamble to rely on clinical instructors and clinics to teach the business side of PT.

As a clinical instructor who takes several PT students every year, I know that PT student are lacking education about PT as a business. PT school teaches you how to become a PT and treat patients. Treating patients, providing education, interventions, and relating to people is a must for all therapists but being a smart business person is a must also. PT schools can do a better job with teaching about insurances, running a successful PT business, and billing and coding. If they do not have a dedicated class on it, then they should bring in guest speakers or people that can talk about real clinic situations and provide an outside perspective from the PT school.

Every PT program will have pros and cons. Strong professors and weak professors. No matter if you go to the highest rated PT school or a middle of the road PT school; they are pretty similar to each other. PT professors will range from great teachers but bad clinicians and vice versa. The best thing a PT student can do is to communicate with a professor pretty regularly, either through class time or office hours. Regular communication with your PT faculty is essential to facilitate learning and will help resolve any and all problems that may arise. You do not want to let any problems go unresolved and for tension and resentment to build up over something that could be resolved quickly. Every student will have trying times with classes, professors, curriculum, and other classmates. Problems with arise and that is part of life but you must try to resolve all issues and problems before they get too big and there is no way for resolution. Talking with your advisor, fellow classmates, and your professors is the best way to get things resolved and for all PT students to reach their maximum potential.

Before PT students hit the job market, they need to pass the national board exam to obtain a license to practice physical therapy in the U.S. Hopefully every PT school gets their students ready to take the board exam and pass their first time but I am not sure that all 200+ schools do. In order to pass the board exam you must take weeks to study with friends, by yourself, and make it your job to focus on the material that will be on the exam. You can use the material that you learned in PT school as a reference but you will ultimately want to use a PT board exam review book. The best source to have for the PT exam is the O'Sullivan review book. You can use Google to find it. It is a great source and is inclusive of all the material needed to pass the board exam.

A great piece of advice that I give new PT graduates is to enjoy some time off before starting your PT career. After you pass your board exam and become licensed, try to take a week or so before you start your first job. Once you start your PT career it is tough to get time off as you will be the low man on the totem pole and most likely working around the holidays. If you have a job lined up and pass your board exam then there is definitely minimal pressure on you after that. Take a week or longer vacation. You were in PT school for 3 long years and stressed out for most of those years. I took my board exam the end of July and passed it my first try so I had a job, a license, and had the rest of my PT career to make money. I filled out the paperwork for my first job but made my start date August 9th and that gave me about 2 weeks to have some fun and go to my brother's wedding before starting my PT career in outpatient orthopedics. Unless making money right away is a priority then enjoy some vacation time before you start your PT career.

Chapter 3

The Costs of PT School

Physical therapy school is an exciting, fun filled, stressful experience that costs thousands of dollars. Three years of physical therapy school will cost most students on average $150,000 dollars. Most students will take out loans to pay for the majority of the expenses they will have to pay over their 3 year PT school experience. If not managed correctly, student loans can cripple a new therapist's financial future. PT school is expensive and a plan needs to be made for repaying student loans and how much money you will need to borrow in order to pay your tuition, living expenses, books, and miscellaneous bills and fees.

Tuition will be one of the biggest expenses a PT student will have to pay every year. Every PT school will have a different price for tuition, so make sure you compare PT school tuition when evaluating which PT school is best for you. Tuition will vary from each of the 200+ PT programs in the United States. There is no set PT program price, so make sure you can afford the PT school however you plan on paying for it. Tuition can range from the low end of $20,000 a year to the high end of around $34,000 a year. A difference of around $10,000 a year for tuition multiplied by 3 years will add up to around $30,000 dollars difference between PT programs. That is a huge difference and must be considered when evaluated PT programs and their costs.

Besides PT school tuition, books, and schools fees, you have to factor in living expenses. Living expenses can range from very minimal if you live at home, to very expensive if you live alone, and everything in between. Living expenses need to be enough to have a safe clean environment without living above your means. There is a fine line between having a comfortable lifestyle to living above your means. A budget for all your bills and expenses needs to be formulated and upheld for every conceivable cost while in PT school.

Knowing your expenses and making a budget while in PT school will ease the stress of managing your money and knowing how much money you will need to borrow with student loans. I wish I made a budget prior to going in to PT school so I would know how much money to save and put aside for my future PT school expenses. Developing a plan is usually a good idea in order to achieve success in all areas of life but definitely one for achieving financial success and growth. You need to know all areas that will cost you money. The cost of living will vary throughout the different areas of the country, so you must budget your specific cost of living for where you will be attending PT school. Listed below is a breakdown of the expenses and costs for the PT school that I attended:

Application Fee:	$50
Acceptance Fee:	$1,000
Health Division Fee:	$145 x 3 =$435
Student Fee:	$945 x 3 = $2835
Annual Tuition:	$26,670 x 3 =$80,010

Additional Expenses
Books, Supplies:	$7500 x 3 = $22,500
Living :	$ 13,000 x 3 = $39,000
Total:	$145,830

NSU, which is located in south Florida, says to budget $13,000 a year for living expenses but I think it will be closer to

$18,000 a year. Even with a roommate to share expenses of rent, utilities, cable and internet, you are cutting it close by only budgeting $1084 a month to live off of. The cost of living in south Florida is very high and you need to budget accordingly. When in doubt over budget your expenses. It is better to plan for higher bills and costs just to make sure that you will have enough money to pay your bills. It is always a good idea to plan for the worst and that is definitely the case with PT school, as PT school bills and living expense can vary each year.

The total bill for 3 years of PT school bills and living expenses on average will be right around $150,000-$160,000. That is a lot of money, and if you take student loans out for the full amount, you will be paying a lot of money over a 30 year loan payment plan. A 30 year loan payment plan will result in a lot of money lost as a result of paying high interest from loan companies. Saving for grad school needs to stay early and often. Students and their parents need to develop a plan to pay for PT school prior to going to college. Potential PT students need to budget for 7 years of school now. Gone are the days of only going to school for 4 years. A budget needs to be set and upheld to assure that loan money does not cripple your financial future after going to school for 7 years.

Most high school and college students do not know what PT school they want to attend until their senior year or college. There are over 200+ PT schools in the country and each have different fees and tuition costs. My advice is to make a list of the top 5 PT schools that you or your child may potentially attend and budget for the highest school on that list. In Florida, there at 10 different PT schools and each have a different tuition costs. The difference can be around $7,000 dollars difference in price each year, which will account for $21,000 dollar difference over the 3 years. Obviously that difference in price should equal better education and teaching but that is not always the case. Physical therapy is a medical field that will only cover so much information. The most expensive PT program should have a better curriculum and staff but that is not always the case. The highest tuition PT programs have similar PT pass rate percentage as the middle of the road PT programs. Now with all that being said, you get what you pay for with most things in life and PT schools is one of them. I do not recommend going to the cheapest PT programs with the worst graduation and national board exam pass rates. I do recommend going to a cheaper school rather than an expensive school. Of the 200+ PT schools, you must find the right program that will provide quality education, information and preparation for the right price. Finding the right PT program for the right price will be a difficult task and needs to be a priority once you think PT is the career for yourself. PT is a great career choice but will cost you a lot of money. I feel that the career will outweigh the costs of PT school but you must develop a plan to pay for it. With the right financial plan that works for you and managing your costs correctly, you can be a great therapist and avoid becoming crippled by the financial debt of PT school.

So many of my physical therapy colleagues plan on getting out of PT school debt when then they are in their 50s or 60s. That sounds crazy and is something that I do not want to be a part of. Knowing that you have a PT school sized mortgage payment along with all your other bills will be very stressful. Expense planning can never start to early, so please start a plan today and become educated of possible PT costs and bills. It will make your life easier down the road and make sure you do not become financially crippled from PT school debt and high interest student loans.

Chapter 4

How to Manage the Costs of PT School

The costs of PT school will result in thousands of dollars in bills and expenses, and the need to develop a budget in order to make ends meet. No matter what PT school you go to and what state you live in, you will have to manage your costs and expenses. Unless you are a millionaire or your parents are paying for PT school, then you will have to think about your money and expenses. The key word there is to "think" about them, do not stress and worry about it but merely think about them and develop a plan on how to pay them back and not live above your means. There are a lot of different ways to manage the costs of PT school and cut your expenses down to manageable levels. By using the tips, strategies, and methods in this chapter you will be able to effectively manage your costs, expenses, PT school bills, and stay within your financial budget.

Did you know that are loan repayment programs and scholarships that are designed specifically for PT students and new graduate PT licensed professionals? Most people do not know about PT scholarships, loan forgiveness programs, and tuition assistance or repayment programs. There are many scholarships through the American Physical Therapy Association (APTA) and other foundations. Scholarships are available for both physical therapist (PT) and physical therapist assistant (PTA) students. Scholarships will vary from the total amount awarded ($1,000-$15,000) to who can win them. The Mary McMillan Scholarship, Florence P Kendall Doctoral Scholarship, and the Promotion of Doctors Studies I & II (PODS) are a couple of the scholarships available to first to third year PT and PTA students. For more information about scholarships and programs please go to http://www.apta.org/CurrentStudents/ScholarshipsAwards/.

PT debt is a part of going to PT school, but there are more and more programs that are offered to help repay your loans and offer loan forgiveness. There are various federal, state, and local programs that are offered now to new graduate PT students. The Indian Health Service Student Loan Repayment Opportunity, Faculty Loan Repayment Program, Public Service Loan Forgiveness, and the National Institutes of Health are a couple programs that are out there that most PT students and licensed PTs do not know about. For more information and details please perform a search on the internet for federal loan forgiveness and repayment programs.

Debt of PT school is unavoidable for most students but how much debt is the controllable factor for most students. PT schools will vary in price so that is the biggest way to control your debt and expenses. If you are already in PT school then knowing the prices of PT schools will not help you, but if you are looking to go to PT school then you need to see the price differences for the PT schools that you are looking at attending. I know in the state of Florida, there are 10 different PT schools and they each vary in tuition price. I went to a higher priced school which cost around 26k a year for tuition, but that was definitely not the most expensive. Florida PT schools cost anywhere from 22K – 33k a year for tuition. That price difference can make a big difference over 3 years. Being in debt even 5k more a year results in 15k over a 3 year program. Potential PT students need to start with calculating the total amount of debt that will be accrued over the 3 years of PT school. The cost of your PT school, living expenses, books, and miscellaneous fees need to be calculated in order to develop a reimbursement plan and know how much debt you will be up against.

Saving your money or cutting your expenses down are the best options for proper management of your money. Having a roommate to split your costs of rent, utilities, electric, cable and internet is one the best ways to cut your living expenses in half. Finding the right roommate may be the difficult part, but once that is done then living together can be fun and a great way to save your money. Maybe you find a roommate that is a fellow PT student or medical student. Finding someone who has a similar schedule and school experience is extremely important. By having similar schedules you can cut your energy bills down and maintain low utility costs. If you have a fellow PT student roommate, then you could possibly cut costs on books, PT supplies, and miscellaneous items that you may be able to share and borrow from each other. PT books are very expensive and if you can share the costs and each buy a book or two instead of each buying all the books from the curriculum, than you will save a lot of money each semester and throughout the PT program. Even if you live by yourself your first year of PT school, as you are new to the area and do not know anyone, you can find a roommate for your 2nd and 3rd year of the PT program. Finding the right roommate may take time so plan on getting a roommate your last 2 years of your PT program as you have to find the right person to life with. People with have different personalities and like to maintain different living situations. Living alone is better than living with a bad roommate, so be patient in finding the right roommate for yourself and situation.

Most students do not live with their parents or close enough to benefit from their free meals and laundry services. I knew a couple PT students that lived at home with their parents while in PT school. They had to drive about 45- 60 minutes to get to school but saved a lot of money by living with their parents. The students did not have to pay rent, utilities, cable, internet, and only had to pay for some part of their daily food expenses. Living with your parents might sound horrible but it might be better than you think. You are always at school, studying in the library or in your room and will have limited interaction with your family. Even if you have a crazy family that frustrates you, saving thousands of dollars a year is worth the price of living with your crazy family. I did not live with my parents during PT school but moved back to NJ for a 2 month clinical rotation during my final year of PT school. It was a great clinical rotation experience and I saved some money living rent free with my parents for 2 months. My parents cooked for me, I did not have to buy food or really anything while being at home. I left early in the morning and came back late in the day so I was never really there accept for dinner time. My 2 month clinical rotation experience is not the same as living with your parents for the whole 3 year PT school length but similar in some aspects. Living at home may be challenging with the family members you may be around but you will not really be at home that much in part to the demands of PT school and you can save a lot of money on living expenses since you will be living with your parents.

PT school needs to be your main focus for the 3 years that you are attending, but you can work as a part time employee to help pay some bills, have some extra spending money, and be able to buy some PT supplies or books. The concept of "earn why you learn" is one that can be considered while in PT school. I worked at the NSU school gym my 2nd and 3rd year as a part time employee for about 20 hours a week. I mostly worked weekends as that was the best time for working hours and did not interfere with my PT studies. Working 20 hours a week and making around 10 bucks an hour will help pay some bills and cut some of the costs of PT school. A part time job needs to be a basic job that will not interfere with your PT school education, curriculum, and studying. It is not worth earning a couple 100 bucks a week if the part time job limits your learning and PT school education. A part time job or seasonal job, if you have summers off or enough time during winter break, should be an option to consider to help manage your bills, living expenses, and PT school costs. A part time job will not make enough money to pay your tuition but should be able to pay your utility bills, a couple books, or some miscellaneous PT school fees that can arise each year.

The best and most logical way to manage your costs is to stay within your budget and to not live above your means. Living above your means can mean a lot of different things to a lot of different people. I see living above your means as spending money that you cannot afford to spend on goods or services that you do not need. PT school costs, living expenses, and any other bills should be documented on an excel spread sheet or paper as to keep track of your expenses and how much money you have available to pay your expenses. Your expenses cannot exceed your budgeted income. Do not pay for elective goods or services (Starbucks, computers, televisions, video games, alcohol, supplements, phones, etc.) unless your money is budgeted for them and you can actually pay for them. Everyone likes to have nice things, but if you cannot afford them then they will have to wait until you have the money to pay for them. Barring unexpected life emergencies (car trouble, medical bills, medication) your expenses need to be documented and budget for. Some people may love the aspect of a budget while others do not like the aspect of being limited and restricted to what they can and cannot purchase. I was the budget person while in PT school. I had fun and a lot of great experiences while in PT school, but made a budget, worked part time, and saved my money in order to buy things and go out to bars and night clubs. I did not live above my means but still had fun and spent money on things that I knew that I could afford.

My friend on the other hand was all about spending his loan money as soon as he got it in his checking account. He bought a new car, a laptop, and even a dog. He owed $200,000 in student loan money from his undergraduate study and probably around

$150,000 for his PT school education. Living it up in college and graduate school is fun but will cost a lot of money in fees and interest when the fun is over. I would rather have some fun during my college and graduate school years but enjoy a house, a nice car, and be able to go on great vacations as a working PT.

When taking out student loan money to pay for your PT school, living expenses, and other bills, you can decide how much to take out. If your loan money is more than you bills, that is fine but do not think of it as free money. Keep that extra money in your account and budget that extra money as an overage and think about taking out less money for your 2nd and 3rd years of PT school. If you have leftover money in your account, then just be smart with the money and plan on doing something positive with the money. I would recommend keeping the extra money in your account for unexpected costs (car trouble, medical bills) as they will show up over time. Having a plan for unexpected bills is always a good idea as they will undoubtedly happen at some point. Your loan money is your income and you need to manage your income wisely as you will only have so much of it while in PT school. Most student loans are paid to students in big chunks 2-3 times a year and those big checks can be misleading to students as they may give a false sense of how much money you truly have. Knowing your expenses and where your money is currently going or will be going in the future is a necessity for proper money management. When in doubt save your money and check your expenses and budgeted costs, as you will be able to pay for elective purchases when you are making the big bucks as a licensed PT but will not be able to become a licensed PT if you do not manage your bills and expenses correctly prior to your completion of PT school.

Chapter 5

The PT Board Exam

The PT board exam is one of the most stressful tests a PT student will take. You have been in school for 7 years and your career cannot start until you pass this 250 question test. I remember taking the board exam and being nervous about passing but felt that I was ready to the take the test after studying for 6 weeks. With the right tools, review books, and study groups you can pass the board exam on your first try.

You will need to buy a national board exam review book. The O'Sullivan Review book for the PT board exam is a great tool and will prepare you for the exam material and format. It is necessary to prepare for the exam through studying the exam material and taking practice tests. The book provides the material that is on the board exam and provides 3 practice tests that will test your knowledge as you study. A review book is necessary to help organize and break up all the material you learned in PT school into several chapters. You can pick up the O'Sullivan review book online (http://www.therapyed.com/ptmain.htm) for $85 bucks plus shipping. That book is a great tool and we highly recommend it for exam prep and getting you prepared for the exam format and material.

Passing the board exam should be taken as your job when you finished PT school and focused on more than anything. Studying every day, meeting with study groups, taking practice tests, and seeking any answers that you might have from fellow students and the faculty of your PT school is what should be done to maximize your studying habits and knowing the material you will be tested on. Along with studying from the review book and meeting with study groups, you can take the O'Sullivan prep course.

The course costs $265 if you bought the review book or $350 if you have not yet bought the review book. The weekend course is ok and provides some strategies for taking the exam. The course is one weekend and will review material from various chapters that you will be tested on. The best and most relevant prep test is the PEAT exam that can be found on the website www.fsbpt.org. The Practice Exam & Assessment Tool (PEAT) is $90 dollars but well worth it. When I was preparing for the exam, I had the O'Sullivan review book, took the O'Sullivan course, and did the PEAT exam. The PEAT exam is by far the most relevant practice test you can take that simulates the real national board exam.

During my last 8 months of PT school we were out of the classroom and into the clinic for clinical rotations. I bought the O'Sullivan review book before my first rotation and studied the material in the book throughout my rotations. I found it helpful to think about the material while treating real patients. I studied the chapters that were relevant for that clinical rotation but really made studying my job right after I graduated. I formed a study group with 2 fellow PT students and we broke up the material into sections, studying 2 sections a week and taking practice tests on Fridays. We met every week for around 4 weeks. We would independently study material from the designated weekly chapters outside of our study group. You have to study alone to see what you know and need to work on. Every day we would study with the group for about 3 hours, answering any questions or problems that we had from the material and practice tests. It was a great way to break up studying, maintaining focus, and retaining the material from the book.

The general format of the board exam is 250 multiple choice questions over 5 hours. You will be able to eliminate 2 choices right away, leaving 2 choices that you will have to pick the best answer to the question. Some of the questions are tricky but you must not over think what the question is asking and only base your answer from the provided information in the question. Of the 250 questions, 50 of them are trial questions and will not be scored. You do not know which 50 are not scored from the bunch so every question counts. Practice tests are the best way to test your knowledge and prepare for the test format. A tip for taking the test is that there is not a penalty for answering a question incorrectly. So you should answer all questions even if unsure of the answer.

In order to get to take the board exam you have to register with the federation of state boards of physical therapy (www.fsbpt.org). On that website you will be able to see the testing dates and what forms need to be sent to your state board. I know in Florida it took about 3-4 weeks to get registered in the system to be able to sit for the exam. The board exam is only administered 4-5 times a year so it is important to register early and find when you want to take the exam. The early bird gets the worm and the PT students who submit their forms early will be able to take the exam when they want to take it.

Besides taking the national board exam, you may have to take a jurisprudence exam to test your knowledge of the state practice acts and laws that are required in the state you will be practicing PT. The jurisprudence exam or law exam as we call it is about 50 questions. The number of questions may have changed, so please consult the website and research how many questions the new test may have. Currently 29 states require a law exam to be taken in order to practice PT, so make sure your state is or is not one of them. Information about the jurisprudence exam can also be found on the www.fsbpt.org website.

Chapter 6

PT Students

Every licensed physical therapist has started their PT career as a student at a physical therapy graduate school. Physical therapy graduates today have a wealth of book knowledge and classroom experience but still lack enough clinical experience to feel very comfortable seeing a lot of patients early on. At any given time there are thousands of PT students from one of 200+ PT schools completing a clinical internship. Of course there are students at varying levels, some are great in some areas and lack in others, while some students might be pretty good at all areas but not great at any specific discipline. Just like in any career or field, there are so many students that have their own strengths and weaknesses. The goal is to maximize your strengths and minimize your weaknesses. That is easier said than done but needs to be done to fully maximize your career potential.

I am a clinical instructor to many students every year that come from many different PT schools. The students vary from different years of PT school and different levels of education. Based on my experiences with students, I have found several areas that most PT students need to improve on. First, most students need to increase their confidence. A lot of students lack confidence with patient interaction, treatment, documentation, and time management. Second, students need to put the process of PT all together from their first encounter with a patient to discharge. Students feel comfortable with performing daily treatments on patients that they have seen several times but are not sure how and when to progress a patient with new exercises and when the patient should be discharged from PT. Third, many students are well educated with classroom information and research based information but cannot bring that wealth of knowledge to patient interaction and treatment on a daily basis. That is no more evident than with documentation and mainly the subjective and assessment portions of the SOAP note format.

Documentation is one of the most important areas in physical therapy. Besides being important to show change over time, what exercises the patient performed, and what your treatment plan is, documentation is important to show any and all discrepancies or problems with patient care. Proper documentation will save your butt against law suits, audits, and patient complaints. Every aspect of the initial evaluation, daily SOAP note, re-evaluation, and discharge are important but the subjective and assessment portions need to be areas of focus and concern. The subjective part is what the patient tells you about how they are doing and how the injury, impairment, and dysfunction are feeling. Students usually have difficulty getting quality information to put in the subjective daily comments due to the fact that the patient did not tell them quality information. Patients usually keep the information short unless they are feeling much better or much worse after their last treatment. When talking with patients you need to ask specific questions about how their condition is doing, if anything is easier to do at home, are they doing their home exercise program, and generally how the body part they are having treated was feeling after last treatment. You can only type what the patient tells you, so you need to ask about every aspect that you can and keep asking questions until they give you quality subjective information.

Some of the best advice I can give a student is that you need to find your own way of being a PT while learning and doing what your professors and clinical instructors tell you. Through your experiences of PT school, clinical rotations, research articles, and just common sense, you can be the PT that you want to be. A PT and even a PT student can have a patient do any exercise that they see fit. As long as you know why you are making a patient do a specific treatment then you can make informed decisions on what is best for the patient. For example, why are you doing that special test, therapeutic exercise or modality with a patient? A lot of PT students know how to perform exercises and activities but are not sure why they should do them and how to progress a patient's treatment. The sooner you understand why to do something with a patient the better you will be as a therapist. There are hundreds of special tests and thousands of exercises to perform with patients and you need to know which ones are best for your patients and why. Understanding pathologies and treatments and ultimately putting it all together comes with experience, clinical decision making, and clinical reasoning.

The field of physical therapy can be an overwhelming experience if you let it overwhelm you and think about every aspect of physical therapy. A great way to understand physical therapy is to break it down into parts. If you break the experience of PT into parts then you can focus on areas of weakness and turn your weaknesses into strengths. Basically PT can be broken down into several parts. You have the initial evaluation, documentation of the initial evaluation, daily treatments, daily treatment notes, re-evaluations, patient care, management, education, and discharge. PT students usually are taught PT in sections of PT and do not get a chance to put it all together. You learn anatomy, physiology, various musculoskeletal sections, specific areas of PT such as cardiopulmonary, integumentary, pediatric, clinical skills, and several neurological courses. There is no course that teaches you the process of how to perform patient care and treatment from a patient initial evaluation to discharge. Putting it all together from initial evaluation to discharge takes time, experience, practice, and education. It is not a quick process by any means.

Chapter 7

Putting It All Together

One of the biggest areas students struggle with is developing and implementing a patient specific plan of care from their initial evaluation to their final discharge. Students feel very comfortable treating patients that they have seen before and have built a connection with. Most students do not know when it is time to discharge someone from PT or progress to harder exercises. It takes time, experience, trial and error, and years of building your knowledge and confidence.

A great way to build your confidence with treating patients for new grads and students is to break the aspects of PT into parts. First is the initial evaluation of any patient for any body part. You need to get proficient at evaluating all body parts of the human body in a 30 minute window. I always try to perform an evaluation along with some treatment and a home exercise program (HEP) within the 1 hour time slot. That can only be done if you have proper time management. If you are not careful, an evaluation can take an hour or even longer. Based on your findings from the evaluation you will develop a patient specific plan of care for that patient. For the rest of that time you need to stay within that plan of care parameters until they are discharged or another plan of care is generated from a re-evaluation. It is very important to put all the planned exercises, modalities, education, activities, and everything that you might perform on the patient in the plan of care. The plan of care can be as simple as therapeutic exercise, therapeutic activities, ROM, which modalities you will be using, and any other specifics.

Goals are generated from the initial evaluation and re-assessed throughout the patient visits. The goals should be functional, measurable, and achievable. Please do not make goals like running 10 miles, 10 box jumps on a 10 inch tall box, or anything athletic unless you are treating an Olympic athlete, professional athlete, or someone that is super high level. Most of the goals should be functional and measurable and simple as increase MMT strength to a certain value, improve functional reach or Apley's scratch test to a specific spine segment, improved squat ability with minimal or no genu valgum, or improve functional gait pattern to normal with normal gait kinematics. When most of or all the goals are met then the patient is ready to be discharged.

Discharge should be thought of from the first day that you evaluate a patient. Discharge is not always a simple task sometimes. In a perfect world, all your patients would get better, improve their function, and have minimal or even no pain or symptoms at the end their PT treatment. That definitely is not the case and should be remembered with some of your patients. Some patients come in with chronic pain, symptoms, and dysfunctions that may not be improved with PT. For those patients, a discharge due to a plateau of progress will most likely be the case. Discharges will be due to many different reasons but ultimately a discharge needs to be done due to medical necessity not being present anymore. Medical necessity is determined for each individual patient that comes to PT. Medical necessity needs to be shown and documented in order to show a basis for continued treatment after the initial evaluation. Sometimes a patient is not a candidate for PT and will be discharged from PT after their initial evaluation based on not showing medical necessity of care. When patients reach a plateau of progress towards PT goals they no longer show a medical necessity and should be discharged as a result.

If all else fails during an initial evaluation, daily visit, or any patient interaction you can treat impairments, dysfunctions, muscular imbalances and anything else that you find that may be a problem. When you treat thousands of patients each year, you will definitely run into tough cases, diagnoses, and patients. For a lot of patients you will not be able to fix their pain, symptoms, and impairments totally with a 100% success rate. Making your patients feel better while increasing their functional strength, mobility, and activity is the name of the game. Being open minded and developing a specific treatment plan for each individual patient is a great way to achieve great outcomes and patient care for all of your patients no matter how hard the case or diagnose might be.

When I treat patients, I like to think about 5 exercises that will effectively recruit each muscle or muscle that I am trying to exercise. By doing that, I have options on what my patient can do. I might have to start light by working the quads with an isometric quad set or maybe they are more advanced and a lateral step down or leg press is what that patient can benefit from. Having options and knowing how to progress and adapt exercises is very important when treating patients. Based on how the patient presents and what functional level they are at after an injury will dictate what your plan should be for that specific patient. Not every patient is created equal and having a mental catalog of exercises for each pathology/diagnosis will provide a therapist with treatment options that can be designed for each specific patient. Once you develop a patient specific plan of care and discover problems and impairments to focus on with the patient, it is your job through interventions, education, and information to get the patient better, stronger, and increasing their function. Simply put, you have to be the one to get the best out of the patient by any means necessary.

Chapter 8

PT Salary

One of the biggest areas that students and new graduate PTs are unaware about is the PT salary. Fair market value of the PT salary is what everyone wants to know about and ultimately get paid. Now your salary will vary based on your location, prior experiences, the cost of living in your state, the type of setting you will be working in, and who your employer is.

Generally you can expect to make around 55k to 70k as a new graduate from PT school depending on what state and PT setting you will be working in. You need to know the base salary for the setting you are going into and the state you will be practicing in. For example, my first job was as a staff PT in south Florida in an outpatient orthopedic clinic and expected to make around 60k as a new graduate. South Florida has a high cost of living which increased my annual salary accordingly. I transferred from southern Florida to central Florida but worked for the same company. My salary remained the same as I transferred within the company that I started with. I am glad that I started in south Florida because I gained around 5k to 6k more working in south Florida vs. central Florida. As you can see, salary will vary even in the same state and setting.

To make the most money in PT, the best areas to work are in a skilled nursing facilities (SNF) or be a travel contract PT that works for 13 weeks at time under a contracted rate. SNF's follow a different reimbursement pay rate than outpatient clinics and hospital settings, so they can pay their therapists more money because the company makes more money. A travel PT has a contract rate that can sometimes pay around 45 dollars an hour, plus travel expenses, living stipends, and other areas of payment.

Most people only care about a high salary and want the most money that they can make each pay check. Some companies might give a little less salary but give better benefits such as chances for bonuses, tuition reimbursement, CEU credits, benefits, Paid Time Off (PTO), 401k, life insurance, and various other programs.

As a general rule I would not work for anything less than 30 dollars an hour, benefits, PTO, 401k match plan, bonuses, annual raise opportunities, and CEU reimbursement or courses provided through the company. Do not be afraid to ask for more money upfront during an interview with a company. If you are worth a higher salary and can/will generate a lot of revenue for the employer then they can usually justify giving a couple more thousand to your annual salary. I asked for a couple more thousand during my initial interview process because I felt I was worth it. Salaries are very negotiable and you should negotiate within reason. Please do not ask for 70k to 80k as a newly licensed PT graduate. I would probably not hire someone if they worried about salary that much and are asking for salary that high. Only bring up the salary if they have not told you about it during the interview process or you feel that the salary is pretty low for the job, like 50k or even 55k in some parts of the country.

A good way to start looking for what fair market value is for your state and setting is to go online to career websites (monster.com, careerbuilder.com) and put in physical therapy and your zip code. There you will get a decent idea of what companies are actually paying. You will be able to see a lot of jobs and compare what companies are offering. You might not take any of those jobs but you can gain valuable information about what the job market is looking like in your desired location.

When we hire a new therapist, we account to make at least 3-4x your salary in gross profit each year. So if you are hired with a high starting salary then you will be expected to earn a lot of revenue for the company. The company needs to turn a high profit on you, plus pay your health insurance, short term and long term disability, PTO, 401k, tuition reimbursement, and any other programs that they might have. A lot of PT companies have the mindset that you need to "earn your keep" to keep your job. Earning your keep is achieved by seeing a lot of patients and making a lot of money while doing it. If you know how to make money treating patients, proper billing and coding, and having a productivity standard of 1.5 patients per hour then you will have no problem staying busy, productive, and be an asset to any PT company or your own business.

Some companies, although very few PT companies, will pay a therapist a flat rate for every patient that they see. A few PTs that I know worked for a company that paid the therapist around 20 bucks for every patient that they saw. The therapists loved it and hated it at the same time. When you were busy you could make a lot of money and when you were slow you barely made money. It would be great making 40 bucks an hour treating two patients an hour. At the same time you may hate that format if your schedule was full of cancelled patients. That model works great when you are busy and it gives therapists incentives to stay busy but a therapist can only do that for so long unless they love the flexibility of the schedule. Again, that model is very uncommon but thought to mention it as it is an option.

Chapter 9

PT Jobs

Physical therapy is a great occupation that provides a sense of purpose, job flexibility, and is very rewarding both financially and mentally. Now if you are getting into PT for the money than that is great but PT is not one of the highest paying jobs in the medical field. People mostly get into this field to help people, be hands on with patients, and really make a difference in someone's life. Whatever your reason for going into physical therapy is, you will have to accept some aspects of the job that may not be so great.

Not all jobs are created equal, even in the same setting. All hospitals are not the same, outpatient clinics vary based on the staff and management, and SNFs will show great variance. Hopefully you can find a job that you love from the very beginning and will want to stay with that company for the length of your employment. There are so many factors that will impact if a PT job is right for you. Everyone wants different things from a job and you need to find the right fit for what you are looking for.

I have worked for a corporately owned physical therapy company since I graduated from PT school. I started out as a staff PT in south Florida but currently work as a center manager of a clinic in the Tampa Bay area. Since I have always worked for a big physical therapy company I was able to transfer without losing my salary, direct deposit, PTO, benefits, and 401k plan. Being able to switch to other locations was great as I like working for my company but wanted to become a center manger instead of staff PT and was able to do that with moving to another location in Florida.

Outpatient orthopedics is a great area of PT with a lot of job flexibility. A PT can be full time, part time, and prn. You can be full time at one clinic, you can be a full time float, and you can be full time or part time between a couple clinics. Part time status means that you will be working less than 40 hours a week on a regular basis. PRN, which means as needed, is great for people who may work another job or want the flexibility to work when they want to work. I myself like being full time in one clinic with a set 40 hours a week. That lifestyle is not for everyone, and you might want the job flexibility of working when you want to work under the prn or part time status.

I had the opportunity to work for a company that I did an 8 week clinical internship with. It was a great opportunity for me to find a first job that I was already familiar with. I cannot tell you how important that experience was, and was a main factor on what job I have today. By taking a job in a clinic that I was already familiar with, I already knew my boss, the front desk staff, staff therapists, the equipment, and the environment I would be working in. Working with familiar faces, location, and equipment will make life easier for you and will limit how stressful things will be.

My first job was at a clinic that I was already familiar with. My second and current job was the complete opposite. I took a job to become the center manager of a clinic without knowing any of the staff, equipment, area, clinic standards, and work environment. That was a major change being the new kid on the block of a center that had all prior staff that knew each other. At times I definitely felt like an outsider and not welcomed, but that was ok as I was hired to turn the center around and make it productive by any means necessary. I saw both ends of the spectrum with starting a new job and it is a lot easier and less stressful working for a company and clinic that you are familiar with.

Productivity is a major area that will affect your daily work schedule, happiness, and general working ability. Basically, productivity is how many patients an hour a PT is supposed to see. We have a productivity standard of 1.5 patients an hour, which is a weird number but better than being expected to see 2 patients an hour. So basically you are supposed to see 2 patients every hour when you can to make up for the new patient evaluations, patients who have Medicare, and federally funded patients that require one to one care. The 1.5 patient productivity standard can be a bit much at times but overall I feel that it keeps me busy and the days fly by with a busy schedule. Some locations market a one to one productivity standard which is great if your patients show up. For the most part you will always have cancellations and if you have one patient an hour every hour you will most likely have a lot of holes in your daily schedule. Holes in your schedule make the day go by super slow and hurt your productivity numbers and revenue. Every PT will be able to handle a different amount of patients and case load that they are comfortable with treating. You need to know what the productivity standard is with a potential job during your interview. Within our company we have a great variety of therapists that are very comfortable with seeing a different amount of patients, for example we have one PTA who wants to see around 3 patients an hour and another therapist who does not feel comfortable seeing any more than 1-2 patients an hour. With every job, you will have employees that want more work and to stay busy or want less work and only comfortable seeing the bare minimum of patients. That is why it is important for all PT clinics to have a productivity standard across the board that is the same for all employees.

As with any job, your work environment, fellow employees, boss, and patient case load will play a major role of your happiness at work. It is very rare to find a great job with every aspect of the job that a person is happy with. Some people might like their fellow employees and the work environment but not like their boss or vice versa. Some people might like their patients and find the job rewarding but have a hard time getting along with their fellow staff.

Even the best jobs have problems but hopefully the problems are few and minor and the main parts of the job are fun and exciting.

Holiday hours are another aspect of a PT job that most people do not think about when PT is your career. Most people celebrate holidays throughout the year no matter what your beliefs are. Patients and therapists are no different in that aspect but they differ as a therapist needs to be available to treat his patients. It is a simple principle that you need to be open for patients to be able to come to PT. That being said holidays are no different in some jobs. For my job we have off 6 days a year for the major holidays, which are New Year's Day, Memorial Day, 4th of July, Labor Day, Thanksgiving Day, and Christmas Day. You have to work Christmas Eve, Black Friday, and a lot of other federal holiday days unless you take paid time off (PTO). If that is not bad enough only getting 6 days a year off, our market manager and upper management want us to make up the holiday hours that we had off for. For example, if Christmas fell on a Wednesday, then we have to make up the 9 hour work day that we usually work throughout the week. So you basically do not work a day for the holiday but make up the hours in the remaining days of the week. Not all PT companies will do that or even clinics of the same company, so knowing your company holiday hours, schedules, and policies is important.

"The grass is always greener," is a great phrase I like to think about when it comes to finding a new PT job after you have in the same job for several years. I have worked for the same company for over 5 years now and have thought about quitting and looking for another job several times but could not go through with it. As a PT there are tons of different PT settings that are looking to employ PTs in every state, so the lack of PT jobs is not a problem. When times are tough, I had a bad week, my boss is driving me crazy, and my staff is making my life difficult I think about how I can simplify my life and take a step back. Being a manager has its pros and cons and a major con is the amount of responsibility, problem solving, and financial stress put upon you every week of every month of every year. That takes a toll on you, at least it has on me so far, and I do not like to get stressed out on a regular basis in any part of my life especially with my job.

I get calls all the time from travel PT companies and emails from local PT businesses looking to hire physical therapists. I have never answered the emails or phone calls to see the specifics of the job but I do wonder what it would be like working for a different company. Working for the same company for over 5+ years has been a great accomplishment and experience, but it is all I know. People are creatures of habit and working for the same company and same clinic is my daily work environment habitat. A part of me thinks about getting a new exciting job with better pay and better hours but remain skeptical that there is a better job for me. What if I leave my current job for a job that turns about to be worse? I have no guarantee that a new job will be better than my current job even if the new job is better on paper with better pay and hours. The work environment could be worse and the staff and I could have total different mindsets.

We all want better hours and more pay and I think working for the same company is the best way to accomplish that. If you start with a new company or clinic, you will be the new guy on the block and most likely be the low man on the totem pole with minimal to no seniority. That being said, you could also be a new fresh face who is a great addition to the team and who has higher productivity standards than the clinic usually has. That is why if you are looking for a new job it is important to know the productivity standards, expectations, and job demands. If you are thinking about leaving your job for a new position or new company, please do a thorough analysis of all the pros and cons. If you are on the fence about leaving but are not sure, try to have a meeting with your boss, if they are open to it, and tell him some of your concerns and feelings about your job and position. Some people of upper management are easy going and willing to make changes to keep their staff happy. While others might take offense to the meeting, so please know how your boss is and judge accordingly. Open communication is a must and saying, "Well I never knew that" or "You never told me" are not acceptable excuses and meetings and measures should be taken to prevent a miscommunication or any problems at work. If you are a good hard-working employee but feel frustrated with your position, responsibilities, or aspects of the job then you should stand up for yourself and talk with your boss about it or start looking for a new job.

There are hundreds of different PT jobs in various locations, states, and settings. Not all PT jobs are created equal and not every PT clinic will be the same. I work in the Tampa Bay area and in our region alone we have 9 different outpatient centers. Each center has different staff, different front desk employees, and a different center manager. My clinic is one of over 900 clinics that the company owns. With that many clinics there is going to be different mindsets of the staff and management. Through trial and error, making connections in the PT world, and doing your homework about facilities, you will be able to find the right job for you and have a long, fun-filled, and rewarding PT career.

Chapter 10

Work Environment

 Work Environment is one of the most important aspects for a therapist to be successful and enjoy coming to work every day. Physical therapy is a very open ended career that gives therapists the options to provide exercises and activities that they want to do. That being said some clinics do things certain ways and maybe that is not what you want in a PT clinic that you will be working at for years. Maybe the clinic is all about productivity, numbers, and making money and you do not want to worry as much about the business end of PT. There are thousands of therapists in the U.S. let alone the world and not every therapist or company will have the same mindset of physical therapy or goals as you might. You need to find the right fit for what you are looking for in a PT career.

 To be successful and provide the highest quality care that you can, you will need to surround yourself with people who will make you better and will encourage professional growth and education. The best way to test the waters of a possible location is to have done a clinical internship as a student at a facility while in PT school. There you will get a 2 month clinical experience of how the clinic works, how the staff and managers are, how busy the clinic usually is, the productivity standards, and the general day to day working environment. Knowing exactly what you are getting into before you start working is an extremely valuable experience that I took for granted when I started working. I can only imagine doing interviews with a company and not knowing what it is really like, how the staff is, how your boss would be, and really how the clinic runs on a daily basis. That would be extremely stressful and nerve racking before you have the pressure of seeing any patients.

I did a 2 month outpatient orthopedic internship while in school and was employed 3 months after I graduated from PT school by the company that I did an outpatient orthopedic rotation with. I applied for the job knowing that I already like the staff, the work environment and what the clinic was all about. I was lucky to have that opportunity and highly recommend trying to work for a company that you do a clinical internship at. If you unfortunately did not have that opportunity, then it may be a little tough but not impossible to find a great job. You have to find out from local PTs at a clinic or better yet during an interview for a job a couple key pieces. You must find out the productivity standards, how many patients you should see in a day and in an hour, how many people work there, and chances to grow with the company. The answers should give you a good idea of what the clinic and company is all about and if that they are a good fit with you.

Another aspect of work environment that most people don't think about when interviewing for a job is your fellow work staff. There are thousands of therapists working today which have various levels of education, certifications, motivation and experience. Some therapists might feel threatened by a new hire and especially a new doctorate of physical therapy graduate. What if you are a new hire and you will be working with veteran staff PTs that have masters of physical therapy and years of experience? They could think, "I'm not going to let some new grad tell me what to do" or "Let's overwork the new hire and see what he has." The new staff might rub you the wrong way or might not respect you early on. People with experience and years at a job get comfortable in a clinic and do not want some new hire messing with their setup and work environment. Now that being said, not all jobs and veteran PTs will be tough on new hired staff members or will be a pain the butt to work with. Some veteran PTs may love a new staff member and welcome you with open arms and make you feel like part of the team. You just never know what type of atmosphere you will be walking into.

Physical therapy is a place to heal and encourage improvement of function, strength, mobility, and activities of daily living. PT clinics should be inviting and a place that people enjoy coming to. A patient can enjoy coming to your clinic for various reasons and the environment should be one of them. The staff, exercise mats, equipment, music, television, waiting room, and general vibe of a clinic will either attract or detract patients from coming to therapy and staying once they are evaluated as a new patient. Interaction between staff, the cleanliness of the equipment and exercise mats, noise and music of the clinic are subtle things that patients pick up on. The work environment rubs off on patient care and it can only benefit you and your business to provide an environment that people enjoy working in and performing PT as a patient in.

A great work environment consists of the people that work together. I encourage a team approach with the clinic staff and patients. A team is way stronger than an individual and two minds are better than one. Even the best therapists need help. Managers need a good productive staff that makes life easier for them. Running a PT clinic is already tough with all the demands of the job and if a manager is having a tough time with everything including his staff then his staff will have to deal with a stressed out manager, and that is never good. When a team has the same goal then they usually work well to achieve that goal. The same mindset goes for a PT clinic. If everyone on board wants to do well, treat a lot of patients, make a lot of money, and make people better than life is usually good. If you have some non-team players and a staff member that does not want what the manager and the team wants then there are bound to be problems and conflicts.

Chapter 11

Find your Niche

Any good business model or company provides a quality service or product that their competitors cannot. The same goes for outpatient orthopedic physical therapy. There are a lot of PT clinics that employ a lot of therapists, so you and your company need to stand out from the crowd. That can be done in a variety of ways some being simple and some not so simple. An easy way to be different then local clinics is to have hours that your patients can come before work, after work, and after school. Being open from 7am to 7pm a couple days a week is a great way to provide hours that will make patients open and available to receive PT. The average person works from 9-5, so being open at 7AM is great for some as they can go to work after PT in the morning or staying open later, after 5PM, so patients can come after work.

Another way to stand out is to provide services that other local clinics do not have. The best services are occupational/hand therapy, pre-employment testing, back schools/programs, vestibular rehab, gait and balance rehab, physical reconditioning programs/work hardening and women's health. Any of those programs/services will provide extra revenue for your company and most PT clinics or companies will not provide all or even some of those services. The services listed above usually will require certifications, licensing, and education about the subject to show that you are able to provide quality care and service. I guess anyone could say they provide vestibular rehab or balance training but you would want to show any and all certifications of programs such as a certification of achievement through the American institute of balance (AIB) that shows that I passed that course and I know what I am doing.

Occupational Therapy and hand therapy are two similar areas but are a little different. In order to be a certified hand therapist you need to study and pass an exam. Hand therapists are a great asset to have in outpatient orthopedics due to the high number of hand injuries that occur in and out of work on a daily basis. More and more hand surgeons will only refer their patients to certified hand therapists (CHT) so it is a beneficial certification for any and all occupational therapists that want to find a niche and corner their local markets.

One of the most common niche markets/areas of physical therapy is women's health. I do not have that distinction as I am a male and that could get tricky as the bulk of your patients would be women. That being said, some men see a women's health PT for certain conditions following prostate surgery. I have worked with a women's health PT before and saw how it could benefit a center as well as the limitations of having one on staff. A women's health PT can only see one patient an hour in most cases due the limitations of the treatment room size they have in a clinic. You need to have a closed private area for patient privacy. When a therapist can only see one patient an hour they are limited with how many patients they can see in a day, week, and a month. Also with one hour blocks of patients, what can be done when patients cancel, reschedule, or do not show up for their appointments. The salaried employed therapist will get paid regardless if they have a patient or not and the niche market or women's health is fairly slow at times and has only so many referring physicians that will send their patient to PT.

A great way to find a niche in your PT practice is to find doctors that will refer patients to your clinic for certain body parts, injuries, and treatment. At my clinic, certain doctors send us patients that have certain conditions, injuries, and surgeries. For example a doctor might send us all of his ACL patients, while another doctor will send us his ankle injuries, and another doctor will refer all his shoulder surgery patients. The niche would be different for each doctor and referring office, but they all need to trust you and your staff that you will get their patients better and that their patients will enjoy coming to your PT clinic.

Chapter 12

The Business of Physical Therapy

When most new graduates of PT school become licensed physical therapists, one of their main goals of any job is to help patients first and foremost and they do not think about PT as a business. Most people in general do not think of the health field as a business, but medicine/health care is one the biggest businesses in the world. Physical therapy is a small part of a huge health care business, but a business none the less. When you manage a clinic or own your own clinic you will definitely think of physical therapy as a business. Any and all businesses have operation costs, budgets, and the need to stay profitable to survive.

The simple way to think of physical therapy as a business is that PT is the business of improving people's function, strength, mobility, and ability to get around. PT is a health care service where people come to get better, stronger, and improve their function. The therapists are the salesmen and the patients are our valued customers. Some patients will need to be sold on the importance of PT and what it will take to get them better. While others will listen and do what the therapist tells them with no selling needed. The best way to be successful in PT is to treat a lot of patients with quality care and have your patients enjoy coming to PT. That is much easier said than done but should be the standard of your clinic and will ensure success as a business.

Any PT business is successful if you make more money than your costs. Sounds pretty simple right? The principle of making money is easier said than done however. Your net revenue needs to be higher than all your costs in the clinic. The costs of your clinic are anything and everything that costs you money, such as electricity, water, equipment, salaries, benefits, and really anything that the

47

company, business owner, or manager needs to pay for. The net revenue is how much is left over after your bills, salaries, benefits, retirement plan, and time off has been paid. You want to have a lot of leftover money in you net when the bills are paid.

"The customer is always right" is a great slogan that all good businesses follow to some extent and the great businesses truly employ on a daily basis. Physical therapy is a people business and our patients are our customers that buy our service, education, and exercises. Our patients pay us through insurance co-pays, co-insurances; private pay through fee for service, or bills after the insurance has received our PT bills. "The customer is always right" is a slogan that all good PT clinics should implement to be successful. Of course patients will not always be right when it comes to their care as they are not medical professionals and it is the medical professional's job to teach them why they cannot do something. You should want the customer to feel satisfied and happy with the care that they received in PT each and every time you see them.

Now that being said, the costumer is not always right in medicine and in physical therapy if they want treatment or care that is contraindicated for safety reasons. Physical therapist should not provide care and interventions that would jeopardize their careers no matter if the patient demands it to be done or not. Patients make demands or suggestions all the time on what they want and how they think they will improve their care and well-being. We need to hear them and make their suggestions happen in some shape or form or educate them on why their suggestions cannot be satisfied. It could be as simple as not doing the bike on their day of treatment because they are not feeling well that day. You would be a fool not to make that alteration to the daily treatment and show the patient that you are there to listen and help them get better at all costs and want them to enjoy being in therapy. By listening to the patient and adapting the daily care you are showing them a way that they are right and that you will be there to get them better.

Insurances (Medicare, Workers Compensation, Managed Care, Tricare, Federally Funded, HMO, PPO) are a main factor in the growth of your PT business. In America people have a lot of different insurance plans and coverage that will affect the number of visits a patient will be coming to PT for. The fact is that the majority of your revenue, unless you are fee for service based, will be how much you receive from insurances payments and reimbursements. For that main point, insurance reimbursement is why I have not and will not try to open up my own PT business. Every year insurance in the U.S. changes mostly to benefit the insurance companies and not medical practices or their patients. As a PT you need to stay on top of the insurance changes and manage them effectively to maximize revenue and adapt to the changes that the insurance companies make.

Chapter 13

Selling PT

Physical therapy is a business. Every PT setting has to deal with costs, budgets, salaries, and many others aspects that will affect how profitable the business is. A PT business is only as good as the managers, the staff, and the therapists that are hired there. The therapists and staff are the face of the business and the reason why a company will succeed or fail. Staff therapists, the front desk staff, and anyone who interacts with patients should be considered an integral part of having success in any physical therapy setting.

As with any business, success and failure is determined by the workers and managers that work for the business, day in and day out. PT is no different than any other health care business, as it can only be as successful as the amount of patients that are treated and how much is paid for services rendered. Insurance reimbursement, patient co-pays and sales are a big part of how successful a PT setting will be. Most people think selling only pertains to products but services can be sold as well. Physical therapy is a service that patients will choose to buy or not. Times are tough in the world and people have far less disposable income then they use to have. People have co-pays of $40, $50 and even $65 dollars per visit. People do not always see the need for PT and especially if it will cost someone 50 dollars a visit and the doctor wants them to come 3 times a week for 4 weeks. If someone has a 50 dollar co-pay and comes 12 visits that will cost them $600 dollars. Six hundred dollars may not seem like a lot of money for some, but for most people who are on a fixed income $600 dollars is a lot to pay in medical bills and will disrupt their budget.

PT clinics need patients to come to their scheduled visits and receive proper reimbursement for services rendered to be profitable. A clinic is only as a good as the therapists that work there and the patients that they treat. Patients are the life line of all PT clinics. Patients need to be treated and valued like very important paying customers. When patients feel valued and appreciated, they are more likely to come back to PT and listen to what their therapist is telling them. Once a level of trust is established between a patient and their therapist, then the therapist can make a recommendation for the patient to continue with PT and purchase any products that they sell in the clinic.

The art of selling PT services and products needs to be a major focus of all therapists in order to help achieve success in outpatient orthopedics. When people think of selling, they might think of a car salesman who is just trying to get a sale and does not really care about his customers or even a person who is selling products door to door. The art of selling gets a bad rap and is generally thought of negatively. In most areas, dealing with salespeople is annoying and most people do not want to be bothered or hassled to buy something. In physical therapy, patients need to be sold on the importance of continued PT care and treatment as the patient may not see the value in seeing a physical therapist. Some patients feel that seeing a physical therapist means that there is a problem and that they may not want to seek treatment until their pain/symptoms are too much to handle. Patients will give you tons of excuses why they cannot come to PT, and it is your job to combat the excuses and try to make the patient become compliant with PT care.

Assuring patient compliance with PT care will be a tough part of patient care. The best way to make a patient become compliant with PT is to educate them about their condition and what it will take to get them better. Educating and informing your patients about their medical conditions, will make them trust your care and ability to make them better. Once a patient trusts you and what you are telling them, then they will be more likely to continue seeing you, show improved compliance with their home exercise program, and may buy some products that you recommend or even sell in your clinic. If the patient will benefit from a product, service, or anything you recommend and you can provide it to them. Why not sell it to them? There is nothing wrong with making a profit off of the PT care, services, and products that are provided and sold in your clinic. No one says that you have to give your knowledge, service, care, and products away for free but therapists feel that they are being unethical and breaking the law if they charge for products and services. Selling PT products and the benefits of PT is not illegal and should be thought of as smart business. Being profitable, providing quality care and great customer service along with quality products is a sign of smart business and PT care.

The best therapists can only treat the patients that show up for their PT visits. If a patient does not come to PT than the patient cannot get better due to the simple fact that the PT cannot effectively treat them. A good PT understands the fact that they are only as good as the patients they treat but a great PT is proactive about making sure their patients come back to see them. I would rather see a patient once a week for 3-4 weeks rather than only seeing a patient once for the initial evaluation. I like to inform my patients that they have options to come to PT but their MD wants them to come to PT 2-3x a week for 4-6 weeks. I try to get on their side and tell them, "I believe you can benefit from 2x a week instead of 3x a week for 3-4 weeks." By letting them know their options for PT visits, I paint a picture that I am cutting them a break with the amount of visits that they should come to PT for and that we can get them better in less time and with less visits than the MD ordered. The selling of PT in that case was that I sold the fact that I was cutting them a break on the number of PT visits that they will need to use in order to get better. Most patients will like the fact that they can get quality PT care and a deal on the amount of PT visits and costs of PT treatment.

A prime example of how the art of selling pertains to PT is when a patient is at their PT session and inquiries about their PT treatment and future sessions. Patients will question the benefits of PT and if PT will truly get them better. It happens almost every day in some form or fashion and a good therapist will sell the benefits of PT to their patients and what it will take to make them better. The art of selling may not even be if a patient buys an actual product; instead they are "buying in" to your care and the benefits of PT. The transaction is achieved when they schedule future appointments and actually show up for them.

A patient asks, "Will I only be doing the same exercises here that I was given to do at home?" How will you answer that question? Based on your response to that question, you will either build a trust with the patient and they will continue with PT or be done with PT after the session and never come back. Of course you want the patient to come back to PT, so carefully answering the question and selling the benefits of PT is important. For the patients that basically do not want to continue with PT after one visit, I try to educate them on their condition and what it will take to get them better. Most of the time, the best treatment is education and information for all patients but definitely for patients who do not see a benefit of PT. I always sell the point that we will design a specific program for the patient and we will constantly be adding new exercises when they hit milestones or show that their basic exercises are too easy. If a patient feels that they can do everything that they do in a PT clinic at home, then why would they need to come to physical therapy and pay you for your services? Basic exercises need to be sold as a home program and something they can do at home. Patient specific PT care should consist of two parts, a home exercise program that is updated as needed and a program that is performed in the clinic. Your specifically designed exercise program needs to be explained to the patient and upheld. If a patient feels that they are paying for a specific custom plan for them then they are more likely to agree with continuing under your PT care and show good compliance with PT visits.

In our clinic, we sell a variety of products that our patients will use at home for their home exercise programs. Our best seller is the product Biofreeze. Biofreeze is a great product to help alleviate pain and soreness that a patient may be having. It comes in a gel, roll-on, and a spray bottle but we only sell the gel and roll on. We make a small profit from each 3oz or 4oz bottle that we sell, but a little profit is better than no profit. We also sell 5ft lengths of thera-band exercise bands; stretch out straps, pulleys, exercise balls, and exercise putty for occupational therapy patients. We provide quality products at low prices. We do not make a huge profit on the products but we provide quality products that the patient can trust are safe and appropriate for them. People can buy a cheaper product online but they do not know what they are getting and the resistance may be too easy or difficult and the product may be cheaply made and could cause them harm or injury. By providing quality products at reasonable prices, our patients get a good deal on quality PT products and the clinic makes out by making a little profit.

The art of selling should not be thought of as a negative thing but merely a way of trying to get your patients to come to PT and stay once you get them in your clinic. I like to use the phrase of "selling PT" but you are only trying to assure good patient outcomes and compliance with PT visits through education and patient communication. Patients may need to be educated and informed about the benefits of PT. With practice and experience you will develop your own way of "selling PT" and achieve success with your patients and in your clinic.

Chapter 14

Insurances

The healthcare system and medical insurance companies in the U.S. are one of the biggest businesses we have in the world. Every person in the United States at some point in the their lives is treated by a medical professional and uses a medical service of some sort, whether it is at a hospital, doctors office, walk in clinic, or pain management office. Outpatient physical therapy is one of those services that sees thousands of patients each year and usually deals with patients insurance for reimbursement and billing claims.

In the outpatient orthopedic PT setting, we have to verify insurances and see what type of plan a patient has before we can treat the patient. Most physical therapy companies accept a lot of different insurances but not every insurance plan. Poor reimbursement rates or a contracted rate could not be established by the insurance company and PT company are two common reasons why a PT clinic would not accept a patients insurance. It is amazing how much variety there is between different insurance plans under the same healthcare company. Most people have blue cross blue shield (BCBS) under their employer but most BCBS plans vary drastically of how much they will cover and how much the patient will need to pay either by a co-pay or co-insurance. I know my own insurance is through BCBS and they have 5 different plans to choose from which all contain different co-pays and coverage plans.

At the clinic that I run, we see a great variety of insurances. Over half of our patients are covered under the workers compensation insurance, followed by Medicare, HMO/PPO or managed care as we call it, and lastly other federally funded such as Tricare which is a military federally funded plan. To maximize your revenue you need to know how to effectively manage and bill the patients insurances to get the most money along with providing the best care. Now there are a lot of different insurances that a PT clinic will encounter. Medicare, Tricare, BCBS, Amerisure, United Health Care, Humana, Cigna, Aetna, Medrisk, Coventry, and the VA are common insurances that you will see in outpatient orthopedics. The therapist and front desk staff need to know how to manage the schedule for proper billing and coding for insurances along with the best ways to maximize revenue from insurance reimbursement rates.

When I started as a PT I felt the divide between insurances and PT services. After years of practicing as a PT I have change my mindset to one of tolerance between insurances and PT care. Now that is not the case with all insurances but it has improved since I started working as a PT. Insurances when managed right will generate a lot of revenue for yourself and your clinic, especially with workers compensation patients. Workers compensation is not a perfect system by any means, but it is a valuable insurance system that when managed correctly can save the company a lot of expenses and care for its employees along with being a good payer for physical therapy services. As with anything, proper care, treatment, and reimbursement start with the communication of all the involved parties such as the insurance case managers, adjusters, doctors, and patients. If there is constant communication between patients, doctors, insurance case managers, and therapists, then therapy services and a plan of therapy should go smoothly and with minimal problems. A lot of the time you will deal with the same people from workers compensation claims and case managers so it is great to build a trust with them and keep the lines of communication open when dealing with patient compliance issues or problems.

Insurance reimbursement is how a PT clinic will make the majority of its money. It is extremely important that everyone that treats patients and bills out services knows how to maximize revenue. Insurances will reimburse based on a variety of factors. Treatment CPT codes, timed units, and length of treatment times for each exercise/technique performed will need to be considered when treating patients. There is great variance of how insurances will reimburse for PT treatments. I cannot speak for all insurances as they will be different for each state and company. Medicare, Tricare, VA, and other federally funded insurance plans are standardized no matter what state or company you will be working for. HMO, PPO, worker's compensation, and managed care insurances will vary from state to state and company to company. Please consult your clinic manager, billing and coding professional, and/or anyone else that might be in charge of reimbursement for your clinic/company to make sure you are maximizing your revenue through proper billing and coding insurance requirements.

The front desk staff is a very important part of maintaining proper insurance reimbursement, obtaining insurance authorizations, scheduling patients to maximize revenue, and verify all of your patient's insurance plans. Making sure you have a great front desk staff that knows the ins and outs of insurance plans is crucial to being successful in your PT clinic. Most people do not realize but PT is considered a specialty under insurance plans and may require a higher co-pay or co-insurance based on the patient's insurance plan. Patients most likely do not know everything about their insurance plan but with the right staff and obtaining the right authorization, the patient will learn about their insurance plan and know what to expect from their PT bills.

Chapter 15

Medicare

Medicare is the federal government insurance plan that everyone who receives a pay checks pays for. Medicare gets its money from the United States tax payers. Medicare is broken up into Part A and Part B. Part A covers inpatient care in hospitals, skilled nursing facilities, hospice, and some home health care. Part B is how we get reimbursed in outpatient orthopedics. When a condition is medically necessary to seek treatment, then Medicare Part B will cover about 80% of the serviced rendered in PT or OT. Medicare is a health insurance program for people who are 65+ years old, or people who are under the age of 65 with certain disabilities. Under the new Medicare regulations, private PT clinics/practices will have a reimbursement cap of $1,920 with an exception allowance of $3,700 based on medical necessity for 2014. Each year the Medicare cap guidelines and cap exceptions can change so you want to stay up on the current guidelines. The Medicare website www.cms.gov is a great Medicare/Medicaid website that will have the information needed to understand the current guidelines and programs.

Medicare is a great insurance program but it does have some flaws and problems that can make life as a PT difficult. The federal government is making the reimbursement of Medicare harder and harder to achieve with new guidelines and procedures that basically complicate our notes and documentation for billing and coding. When managed correctly, Medicare is a great payer and insurance for a patient to have in PT. Medicare reimburses outpatient orthopedics by time based units. 1 unit = 8-22 minutes, 2 units = 23- 37, 3 units = 38 – 52, 4 units = 53 – 67, 5 units = 68 – 82 minutes. The time based units are extremely important to memorize and know for each and every Medicare patient that you will see. Please know the amount of time that is needed to satisfy 4 quality units of care. Four units is the most common number of units for each hour of care and should be achieved for all Medicare patients.

Medicare is so complicated that you could write an entire book about it. Here I will highlight the main things to help manage your Medicare patients and make the most revenue possible. First and foremost you should never treat a Medicare patient with another patient during the same hour of treatment. By doing that you will have to group the entire time they are treated with the other patient and you will lose a lot of potential profit. The average PT session is 45 to 60 minutes long. If you bill out 53-60 minutes of time based treatment codes then you would get your 4 units of treatment based care for a Medicare patient which would amount to just over 100 dollars for your clinic that hour. If you grouped that hour you would get around $17 dollars for that hour with that patient plus the insurance of the other patient but only $17 for that Medicare patient. In that patient scenario, you would miss out on $83 dollars by grouping Medicare patients. Losing money from improper billing and scheduling is a recipe for disaster and missed revenue. Secondly, are you billing under the appropriate CPT billing codes for the treatments that you performed? The CPT codes are the billing codes that state what the exercises/education that was performed by the patient or therapist on the patient during treatment. For example any and all strengthening, endurance, ROM, and flexibility exercises should be billed as therapeutic exercise which is CPT code 97110. Gait training will fall under gait training 97116, manual therapy such as manual traction, joint mobilizations, and soft tissue techniques are under 97140, all work related duties are therapeutic activities 97530, and balance, proprioception, posture, and coordination should be billed as neuromuscular re-education which is code 97112. Thirdly and most importantly you need to keep all treatments and documentation related to functional deficits and improving their functional strength, mobility, and return to their prior level of function. Your treatment might be functional and goals may be function related but your daily assessment and documentation may not be function related and show medical necessity. If your notes do not show medical necessity, functional deficits, and long term functional goals, then a Medicare auditor can and most likely will refuse payment for services rendered. Which is unacceptable and an hour long waste of time if you did all that treatment/care for no payment. There is nothing more frustrating than doing a lot of work and not getting paid for it.

Another important aspect of treating patients who have Medicare insurance is that you must document a Medicare diagnosis ICD-9 code in your notes and initial evaluation. The ICD-9 code is a code that is internationally recognized by all health care professionals for what body part and dysfunction you are treating. For example it can be as simple as 724.2 Lumbago for lumbar spine pain or 723.1 Cervicalgia for neck pain. There is a big list of commonly used ICD-9 codes and Medicare ICD-9 codes online and in our appendix in the back of this book. Medicare ICD-9 codes can be used for all patients but they must be used for all Medicare patients. If you do not put an accepted Medicare ICD-9 code during your initial evaluation then Medicare can deny payment for services rendered, so as you can see it is very important to have. For a list of common Medicare accepted ICD-9 codes, please consult the appendix in back of this book.

In 2013, Medicare decided to add another requirement in order to receive proper reimbursement with the addition of G-Code modifiers. G-code modifiers are required codes that must be documented during a patient's initial evaluation, re-evaluation, and discharge. G-code modifiers are codes that need to be placed in your documentation that state what current level of a certain activity the patient is at currently and what the goal is for that activity. There are different codes that will be used for documenting the patients current status, goal status, and discharge status, of various activities such as mobility, walking & moving around which is G8978. The different activities have different g-codes and you need to have the same g-code for the current status and goal status. For example you cannot have a mobility g-code of carrying, moving & handling for the initial current status goal and a goal status g-code modifier of mobility, walking and moving around. The two g-codes are not listed under the same categories and will have different sequential numbers. As carrying, moving, & handling object is G8984 where mobility, walking, & moving around is G8978. The g-code needs to be sequential and under the same category. For example if a patient has a shoulder dysfunction then you most likely would use the g-code of G8984 which is carrying, moving, & handling objects at the current status. The goal status g-code would have to be G8985 under the same category of carrying, moving, & handling. The current status g-codes at evaluation would be G8984 followed by the goal status of G8985. The numbers are sequential and are under the same categories. The g-code modifiers can take some time to learn but they need to become second nature to assure that no conflicts will result with Medicare guidelines and to avoid any reimbursement issues.

Chapter 16

Workers Compensation

Workers compensation is an important insurance company that provides care for injured workers who were injured while working on the job. Workers compensation claims are a major source of patient visits to doctors' offices and physical therapy clinics. The bulk of my daily case load in my clinic is mainly workers compensation. About 60 percent of all the patients that we treat at our clinic are sent through various workers compensation insurance companies. We see a lot of workers compensation patients and have learned how to manage them effectively. As with any insurance company, you need to know how to manage the insurance plans to effectively generate the most revenue possible while getting the patient better. The PT treatment goal for every patient is to get them better and return them to their prior level of function. The goal for reimbursement in physical therapy should be to generate the most revenue possible with proper billing, coding, and charging for all patient based on there insurance.

Patients who have workers compensation insurance can be major headaches, show poor compliance with visits and exercises, and for the most part cause therapists undo stress. As with any patient insurance, you need to know how to effectively manage them to fully maximize insurance reimbursement and have the patient reach their rehab potential. That is definitely easier said than done. I see a lot of workers compensation patients and it is getting tougher and tougher to manage them effectively. Insurance companies are starting to reimburse less money and expect you to get their patients back to work faster. So you are working harder and getting paid less. That is the wrong way of things, people want to work less and get paid more. Not all workers compensation companies are created equal and will reimburse differently however. We see a variety of workers compensation insurances. Johns Eastern, Sedgwick, Alignetworks, Zenith, Coventry, Medrisk, and SPNet are some of the workers compensation insurance companies that we receive patients from. Some of those insurances pay a flat case rate of $65 per visit and other companies will pay based on a fee schedule. The fee schedule is usually 85 percent of what Medicare pays for time based treatment codes. The care that you provide should not change based on the insurance reimbursement but your billing and use of CPT codes may change based on the insurance reimbursement rate.

When possible you want to communicate and build a connection with workers compensation case managers and doctors. Workers compensation patients can be stressful, frustrating, and a major pain in the butt. Constant communication either by phone call or faxed documentation to the MD and case manager is a must to stay on top of non-compliant frustrating patients. All of your patients will come to PT for different reasons and workers compensation patients are notorious for coming to PT for reasons other than to get better and return to work. Proper documentation needs to be performed for all patients but especially for all workers compensation patients. Workers compensation companies send their patients to PT to get them better and have them return to work. If a patient is not taking the steps to improve their function and resume their prior level of job function, than communication with the referring MD and case manager needs to be initiated to discuss continued treatment of the patient. A team approach should be considered when treating workers compensation patients. The team is made up of the patient, MD, case manager, and the physical therapist. The goal of the PT care should be to get them back to full duty status and the patient needs to show consistent effort and compliance with that goal.

Workers compensation patients will generally either be very compliant with PT visits or non-compliant in general. Patients need to know what is expected of them in consideration to PT visits and home exercise programs. Patient ignorance is no excuse for missed visits and general non-compliance with PT. If a patient continually misses PT appointments then the case manager must be notified and most likely a discharge summary will be documented and the patient will be discharged due to patient non-compliance. Before we discharge a patient, either the therapist or front desk staff calls the patient one last time to get them back into PT. If the patient does not answer and/or call us back, then a discharge (D/C) due to non-compliance will be completed and sent to the case manager and the referring physician.

The last thing a therapist wants to do, is to discharge a patient prior to getting them better and achieving their PT goals. Workers compensation patients can test that dilemma on a regular basis. Workers compensation patients can be tough, complex, and frustrating patients. Workers compensation patients will be sent to PT for a variety of diagnosis and injuries but most commonly they are sent for low back, neck, shoulder, and knee injuries. No matter what condition or pathology a patient has come to PT for, your goal is to get them better and back to work.

My experiences with workers compensation doctors and their patients has been one of frustration more than one of pleasure unfortunately. I have seen patients who need surgery but have been sent to PT in place of having surgery. For example, I had a patient who twisted his knee while at work and suffered a major knee injury. The patient was on crutches, could barely put weight on his R leg and could not bend his knee more than 65 degrees without severe pain and symptoms. I knew that his outcome and prognosis in PT were not going to be good unless surgical intervention was performed. The doctor wrote a prescription for 12 total visits and the insurance authorized the 12 visits. It was clear to me that the patient would not make enough progress to return to his prior level of work function and to perform his activities of daily living (ADL) at the same level he did before his injury. I documented my objective findings and my clinical assessment to show that he may benefit from treatment outside of skilled PT to fully maximize his rehab potential and ultimate goal of returning to his prior level of function. This basically meant that I recommend surgery instead of continued PT in order for him to make a full recovery from his injury. My documentation was sent to the MD and case manager to show my recommendations and if the patient was a good candidate for PT. The case manager and doctor said to keep treating the patient and we will re-evaluate the patient after 4 weeks of PT. We saw the patient for 4 weeks and he showed minimal improvement in range of motion, strength, and his ability to walk. He liked coming to PT and wanted to get better but ultimately needed surgery to fix the anatomical dysfunction and injury that he suffered at work. I will never forget how much he suffered while being in PT and saw how the workers compensation company strung him along. After 7 months after his injury, he finally had knee surgery to clean up the knee joint and came back to PT after the surgery was performed. The surgery made his knee less painful but ultimately he could not return to his prior level of work function and was fired from his job. Not to say that if he had the surgery earlier that he would have made a full recovery and still be working that same job, but we will never know since it took 7 months to have surgery after his injury. That is only one case and not what to expect with all patients who are sent from workers compensation but my continual experiences with workers compensation patients have shown that there does not seem to be a rush to get the patients the care that they need as soon as they need it.

Communication with workers compensation case managers and the referring MDs need to be achieved early and often. Even with the consist communication with all parties from workers compensation companies; there will be delays in patient care and the best course of treatment. I am continually frustrated with workers compensation MDs that will keep sending a patient back to PT who has reached a plateau of progress towards PT goals and will no longer benefit from PT care. A doctor outranks a physical therapist and whatever the MD wants for the patient, they get for the patient. Workers compensation is a broken system and will cause you much stress and frustration. All you can do is to accept its flaws and try to get your patients better and document everything that you find, see, and assess. Covering your butt with proper documentation needs to be a standard with all patients but especially for those who are sent to PT on a workers compensation claim. The workers compensation system is a frustrating system that will cause much undo stress and headaches. Therapists need to know how to manage the workers compensation system to benefit them and their clinics. Through experience, time, and connections in the workers compensation system, you will be able to deal with the flaws in the insurance system and maintain a high level of patient care and revenue.

Chapter 17

Documentation

The most important aspect of physical therapy is documentation. If you can document well then you can be a great overall therapist. When I was in physical therapy school, one of my professors always said "If you did not document it, then it never happened." That phrase did not mean a lot to me until I was a licensed PT and saw how documentation could affect my license and career as a therapist. Documentation is a boring tedious process but needs to be a major focus of your day to day patient care to safeguard yourself against law suits and legal measures that a patient may have against the care that you provided.

As a physical therapist you deal with some dicey situations and you need to keep a very good paper trail of all aspects of patient care for every patient that you have treated. You never know when a litigation case needs your notes for their case or if someone has a dispute about the care you gave them. If you have a well-documented paper trail for that patient, then in most cases your notes will get you out of trouble. Proper documentation will save you or hurt you if a law suit or audit of your facility is done, so you have to document everything that goes on during any and all interaction with your patients. Documentation is something that takes time and experience to get good at, and then even after that you still might commit errors or mistakes.

The style of documentation can be unique to each therapist but needs to cover certain topics, contain proper safe verbiage that cannot be construed against you, and paint a picture of how the patient is doing from that day of care and overall since starting PT. Proper verbiage must consist of terms, phrases, and words that are not definite unless they need to be, such as "Discharge patient to

HEP due to completed program." Most of the time you need to be direct and to the point but in a way that is not right or wrong, such as "Patient may be reaching a plateau of progress towards PT goals as evidence by minimal function ROM improvement with functional reach overhead and behind his back." You have to use words like "may" that are not definite and could be construed as one way or another. Not like "will" that is saying that the patient has to have this or that to be better or not.

Functional outcomes are great necessary forms of documentation that need to be done with all patients. Functional outcomes are various forms that ask questions about what the patient can do, how difficult an activity is, and then scored and compared to normative values that were established. The Oswestry, Neck Disability Index (NDI), Lower Extremity Functional Scale (LEFS) and the Shoulder Specific Disability Index (SPADI) are common outcome measures that we use on a daily basis.

More and more companies and PT clinics are making the transition to computerized documentation. I have only had computerized documentation as a licensed PT. It makes your life a lot easier and simplified than paper documentation. That being said, since it is computer based and connected to the internet there can be problems associated with connectivity and server issues. No matter what type of documentation system you use at work, you have to have high standards while performing initial evaluations, progress notes, discharge summaries, and daily SOAP notes.

For those who might not know, but we use the SOAP note format to document. The SOAP note stands for S = Subjective, O = Objective, A = Assessment, and P = Plan. The subjective part means that it came from the patient/subject. The objective part means that it came from the therapist from test and measures such as ROM, MMT, and special tests. The assessment section must come from the therapist and contain information about how the therapist feels the patient is doing in therapy, any impairments and dysfunctions that may remain, and clinical judgment to back up the findings with evidence found by the therapist. The plan part is what you plan on doing with the patient and what exercises, activities, modalities you will be performing throughout their care in PT.

Some samples of proper documentation are listed below:

Subjective

"Patient reports that her lumbar spine dysfunction and pain/sx limit her ability to perform ADLs and basic care at her premorbid status of independent without difficulty"

Patient reports that his R knee is feeling better today, compliance with HEP, and that he can go up and down stairs with less pain now.

Assessment

Pt may be reaching a plateau of progress towards PT goals of increasing functional pain free ROM, strength, flexibility, and stabilization as evidence by the minimal improvement of the ability to perform sit to stand, gait, and therapeutic exercise without moderate difficulty and pain/symptoms.

Pt continues to demo progress towards PT goals of increasing functional strength, pain free ROM, joint mobility, and stabilization with minimal difficulty and pain/symptoms

Plan

Continue focus on increasing L shoulder functional strength, ROM, stabilization, and joint mobility

Chapter 18

Patients & Their Families

Patients want to feel that you are on their side and you want to get them better. Every patient, especially new patients should be greeted with a smile, a handshake, and the general feeling that you are there to get them better at all costs. Ok, that last part might be an exaggeration but they do need to feel that you are on their side and you want them to make a full recovery. Patients are what drive our profession and the reason why people become physical therapists. Now some patients will drive you crazy, they will ask a million questions, they will not agree with what you are doing, and they might even complain to the doctor about you and physical therapy in general. Even after all the negative bad patients that come in the door, your job is worth it when you get that one patient who loves coming to physical therapy and does everything you say. Hopefully your good patients will outweigh your bad patients, but that is part of working with the general public, you never know who you are going to get as a patient. That is why you need to treat all patients fairly, equally, and with the care that you would want done to you.

Patients in physical therapy range from babies to the elderly and everything in between. That being said, you probably would not interact and communicate the same with an elderly women versus a teenage boy. The same goes for treatment plans and goals of PT for each patient. A teenage boy recovering from shoulder surgery should recover faster than an elderly person who suffered the same injury. That should make sense and must be remembered when treating patients. The primary goal for your patients should be to return them to their specific prior level of function, which will be different for each patient and needs to be adjusted accordingly.

A sad but true aspect of physical therapy is that not all patients get better in our care. In a perfect world we would be able to cure all our patients' problems and ailments. I am firm believer when the time is right you need to be the bearer of bad news and be direct but sincere and respectful when delivering bad news to patients. We cannot get rid of every ache and pain that our patients may have. We may not be able to get an 88 year old patient to feel 34 again, but we can improve their function, strength, and general wellness. Some patients will not accept that they are getting older, or that their condition is reaching a plateau and may not get any better than where they currently are. I believe delivering false hope to someone is far worse than telling someone the truth about their condition. Now that does not mean that you have to put the patient down or tell them bad news right away, but you should be realistic with their care and goals. If someone who is 85 years old and has severe degeneration of their shoulder joint, they most likely will not remove all the pain and regain 100% function again. Degeneration of joints and muscles is pretty much an irreversible process and can only be improved so much. You have to develop a way of keeping things positive but realistic for patients. It will be tough to keep things positive for all patients but finding the bright side of things with patients will make your life easier and keep patients positive about their recovery.

The more a patient works with a therapist the more that patient will trust the therapist. The therapist patient connection is a strong bond and tough to break once it is established. When a strong bond is formed patients usually only want to work with the same therapist that they have been seeing since their initial evaluation. We try to keep patients with the same therapist but that cannot always be done. When working with a new patient for the first time that usually sees another therapist, you can expect some hesitation from the patient as you are new to the patient and have not formed a patient therapist bound yet. Some patients will refuse to work with someone new for fear of inferior treatment or having to start over with someone new. Do not get frustrated or take offense to that, as the patient usually just wants to work with their familiar therapist regardless of who you are. In fact you could be a new, exciting, and fun PT that would be able to help the patient but the patient does not know that and it is your job to build that connection and trust with the patient. A great way to cut the tension when starting with a new patient is to say, "Hi, my name is Brian and I will be working with you today, I got special instructions from your previous therapist (say their therapist name) about what is going on and what we should work on." By doing that they will know that you are working together with their previous therapist and you have a plan. Building trust with all patients whether they are new or not should be focused on and achieved quickly. If the patient is defensive to what you are telling them, then they will have limited beneficial results in PT.

The "Power of Positivity" is a great concept that should be done with every patient no matter how difficult it might be. No one likes to hear bad news especially when it comes to their health. Not every patient does better in PT but every patient should feel that they are getting better in some form or fashion. When you ask patients about how they are feeling or if anything is easier to do at home, try to bring out some activity that may be easier to perform or that they could not do before. When someone is walking better or showing signs of improved function, make it a point to tell the patient that they are doing better and that they're walking better or doing an activity now that you know they were not doing the first day you saw them. Staying positive can be as easy as saying that someone is doing an exercise correctly or their form is looking good. For the patients that actually tell you that they are feeling better and getting around easier the positivity is easy and coming from the patient. The patients that are always negative and tell you that they are about the same or actually worse with PT might be harder to stay positive with. The negative patients will be the ones that you have to find the silver linings for and bring the patients attention to progress of improved function, mobility, or strength. Negative patients will focus on all the negative painful things and might not realize that they may have improved strength, mobility, ROM, and flexibility. With all the being said, no matter what you do with some patients, some patients will always be negative and refuse to show happiness with treatment or progress towards their goals. You can't win them all, but you should want to try to win and open the eyes of all patients about their conditions as you do not know how much a patient is learning from you.

Patients are our customers and they need to be treated and valued like paying customers. Patients are buying your care of physical therapy service. Patients want to feel like they are the only patient you are seeing and treating, even if you are busy with 2 to 3 patients an hour. To get the best result for all your patients, you need to treat under a rule of specificity for each patient. Specificity for each patient means that you don't treat all patients the same. It is very easy to say and extremely hard to do, but if you take your time and develop a patient specific plan of care from the initial evaluation on day one, it is a lot easier. Patients and mainly patient's bodies are definitely not the same so you need to remember that when treating patients with similar injuries. Similar exercises will be done for most patients with the same injured body part but do not turn into a one trick pony and do the same exercises for everyone.

Not all patients are created equal and we need to remember that when treating our patients. You will see a lot of patients as a therapist each day and over your career. It is easy to group all patients with a specific injury into a certain category and perform the same exercises for all. It is easy to develop some biases and tendencies of treatment for patients with common diagnosis that you see every day. For example, you might do the same exercises for patients with low back pain based on your years of experience and training. For the most part that is fine to do but we develop habits and biases that may not always be what is best for our patients and clinic. Some patients will heal faster than others, some will want to push pass the discomfort easier than others, and some patients will need a lot of encouragement and positive feedback to know that they are getting better by the care that you are giving them. Developing specific exercises and adapting treatments based on patient tolerance is vital to success for all patients and must be done.

A great piece of advice when treating patients is to not overestimate or underestimate what a patient can do based on what you think their functional level is. I have learned from experience that a lot of your patients will surprise you. I cannot count how many times I have seen a patient who can barely walk in from the waiting room be able to pedal on the bike for miles, going up and down steps in the parallel bars, and do a leg press with minimal difficulty. Looks can be deceiving and that is definitely true in PT. You have to think about increasing a patient's function safely and effectively no matter what impairments, dysfunctions, symptoms and pain the patients are dealing with.

With years of experience as a licensed PT you will see a great variety of patients. Some patients you will love working with and others you will dread seeing each visit. People have different personalities but as a medical professional you need to put that aside and focus on getting the patient better even if they drive you crazy, ask a million questions, are non-compliant with PT, and just generally make your life harder as a therapist. Your patient population will test your limits, patience, and nerves but that is what makes the job fun and challenging. The best advice I can give when working with tough patients is to have an open mind, stay positive, and have empathy and compassion for all patients. Having empathy and compassion is part of PT and can only help you relate to the patient. Developing a good relationship with difficult patients is tough but needs to be done and can be rewarding when accomplished. I know it will be tough, as I have had to do it first hand, but staying positive, friendly, and nice to your patients will improve their well-being even if they do not tell you it is. Some of the most memorable patients are ones that were a pain in butt, did not want to be in PT, and generally made you crazy every visit. Remember a patient is usually only seen for 1 hour at a time, a couple times a week, for a couple weeks, so at worst you need to grin and bear it for those couple hours a week.

Patients for the most part are great, compliant, and willing do whatever it takes to get better. When you have a good, nice, and hardworking patient, nothing is better in PT. When you have the exact opposite with a patient, live is stressful and irritating. There is nothing worse as a PT when you have a busy day filled with pain in the butt non-compliant patients that show up when they want. They ask you a million questions, don't want to do certain exercises, don't trust what you tell them, and they really don't want to be in therapy. The patient might be even getting better with less pain and more function but they never tell you that and they usually say that they are about the same or still having pain.

Another bad scenario is that a patient cannot keep their appointments; they keep rescheduling and always have an excuse for missing appointments. You want to believe them, so you keep moving them around on the schedule to try and help them but they keep missing appointments. In a situation of patient non-compliance with PT visits, you need to communicate with the patient that missing appointment is not acceptable and needs to change. As you cannot get someone better if they are absent from treatment sessions. However, even with proper communication with patients, they will either show up or not for PT. You can only do so much to assure patient visit compliance but you have to try and that is all you can do.

With any bad patient you have to choose what can be done to remedy the problem and make sure the patient improves their compliance and attitude. Communication and early communication needs to be done to have everyone on the same page. The patient could be ignorant to the fact that there is a problem or that they are doing anything wrong. The expectations and standards of your clinic and care need to be understood by the patient to assure proper compliance with visits, HEP, and treatment. If a patient is told and understands the plan and what is going on with their condition then they are more likely to be compliant and follow through with treatment. By giving the patient the information to get better and what is expected of them in PT, the "ball will be in their court" and they will chose if they are buying into PT or not. You cannot force someone to listen to you or even be compliant with PT but you have to try and that is all you can do. Lack of effort from a PT is unacceptable and not what you go to school for 7 years to do. It will be tough at times and your limits will be tested with those tough patients so expect some conflicts. You need to develop a specific plan on what works for yourself and clinic. Patient interaction is something a PT will develop over time and is essential to success with your patients and growth of your clinic.

Chapter 19

Treating More Than One Patient an Hour

Treating more than one patient an hour is a great way to increase productivity and grow your business. Treating several patients at the same time sounds great on paper, but is much easier said than done. The only way to treat more than one patient an hour efficiently and effectively is with proper time management. Time management is important with every aspect of daily life as a therapist, but is the most important aspect to consider when treating multiple patients during the same hour of treatment.

Patient care should never be compromised when treating one patient or multiple patients. Providing quality care for all patients while completing your documentation and daily tasks in a timely manner needs to be a major priority of every therapist. Even the worst therapist can treat one patient an hour, but the best therapists can see several patients an hour without sacrificing quality of care and documentation standards. Every patient will require different levels of care, cuing, direction, and attention, so it will require some effort to achieve your patient's goals and maximize their rehab potential when treating several patients at once.

Treating several patients an hour can be very stressful and difficult but with the use of several tips and strategies that I have developed firsthand, you will be able to treat several patients an hour with ease. Treating several patients at one time starts with maintaining a productive schedule that accommodates patients but also accommodates the therapist. If possible, you should try to schedule a patient that requires minimal hands-on care and guidance of their exercises with a patient that requires a good amount of manual therapy and attention of the therapist. There you can have a good mix of hands-on treatment and exercise with the two patients. Having two patients that require a lot of manual therapy and hands-on care is difficult to provide quality care to both patients at the same time. So when possible, take control of your schedule and schedule patients at preferred times to maximize patient care. That is much easier said than done and with time and experience it will be easy to say and do.

      The first thing that every therapist must do when treating more than one patient an hour is to have a daily treatment plan for your patients. Each patient needs to feel that they are being treated as if they were the only patient being seen that hour. Bikes, pulleys, treadmills, and arm bikes are necessary to use with patients to provide treatment for one patient as you provide manual therapy hands-on treatment for the other. Since you only have two hands, you can only provide soft tissue manual therapy, passive ROM, joint mobility, and other manual techniques for one patient at a time. As you are busy with one patient you need to find exercises and activities for your other patients to perform while your hands are occupied with the other patient. Simply put, you need to have activities and exercises for each patient that you are treating with minimal to no lull in treatment for each patient. No matter what the patients are being treated for, you need to effectively treat your patients with the appropriate exercises, activities, and techniques. Knowing a staple of exercises for pathologies that you normally treat and how to progress and adjust exercises is important, as you might need to adjust exercises for each patient on the fly. As one patient is performing one exercise, you need to know the next couple of exercises that you will be giving the patient so you can move the patient along without hesitation. Efficiency and time management are important when treating multiple patients at once.

Knowing the exercises that can be performed for your patient's pathologies is a necessity for good therapists to become great therapists. Exercises need to be thought of as the tools that will help treat your patient's pathologies and also help manage patient care when you are treating more than one patient an hour. When treating two exercised based patients an hour, you need to have a patient specific exercise plan for each patient since you will be switching back and forth to each patient giving them new exercises once they have finished an exercise. When one patient is performing an exercise safely on an exercise mat, you can leave that patient and go treat the other patient with another exercise or intervention. You must be able to leave a patient when they are performing an exercise independently to free up your attention to focus on your other patients. That is where knowledge of exercises will benefit a therapist as they can have their patients perform several exercises without delay or hesitation.

Teaching your patients exercises and the PT routine after they have been coming to PT for a couple of visits will make your life a whole lot easier when you are treating more than one patient an hour. After a patient has been coming to PT for a while they will usually know the routine and can complete a lot of their exercises with minimal help or guidance from the therapist. The therapist will supervise the independent patient but spend the bulk of their time with the patients that need more hands-on treatment and guidance. As a physical therapist, you need to learn to divide your time between your patients and tasks. Anything that can be done to ease patient care and time management should be done, as treating more than one can be stressful. Through experience and practice, you will be able to treat several patients an hour with ease and may even become bored with treating only one patient an hour.

Chapter 20

The Schedule

Physical therapy has a very simple business model for success, the more patients you see the more money you make. The schedule is the framework for success or failure. If you have scheduled hours that are not available for patients to come to PT then you will have trouble filling the hours with patients. Typically patients work 9-5 Monday through Friday, so the PT clinic must be open before 9 and after 5 for the general working population. Of course the working population is not your only case load, so being open in the middle of the day or afternoon is usually good for the elderly, people who do not work such as students or workers compensation patients and people that are off from work or have a flexible schedule.

My clinic is open Monday through Friday, is open at seven 3 days a week and closes at seven 3 days a week. Some clinics are open on Saturday mornings to offset shortened hours doing the week. Unless you own a business, the general work week for full time employees is 32-40 hours to be classified as a full time employee. 40 hours a week can be scheduled anyway you want but should be set to maximize patient care and visits. The schedule and hours should be set to see the most patients and therefore maximize revenue. If you clinic is not as successful as you would want it to be, first take a look at your busiest hours for patient care and try to stay open around those hours and if possible hire more people for that time.

The schedule is what can drive you crazy or make you happy. Some of the busiest days as a therapist are when your schedule is full and the patients show up for their appointments. The schedule will have limitations for growth and productivity but it must be managed well and appropriately to maximize revenue. The biggest culprit is with Medicare and other one to one scheduled patients. Remember the best way to make the most money is to have more people schedule during one hour of work. Medicare and federally funded patients must be schedule alone during an hour to maximize revenue. If a Medicare is grouped with another patient during an hour treatment you must bill a group charge and will lose around $85 dollars by grouping instead of billing out 4 quality individual units versus 1 group charge. If you don't have a Medicare patient or one to one patient you can load that hour on your schedule up with as many patients as you can handle. Now that being said, if you have too many patients each hour they will most likely receive poor quality care since you have to split your time between several patients instead of one on one care. A happy medium must be established for each therapist and that usually depends on the patients being scheduled each hour and if they require a lot of manual therapy, exercises, and therapist interaction. The best hour of a therapist schedule besides the last hour of the day is a busy mix of independent exercise patients that require some manual therapy, education, and patient-therapist interaction. The hour will fly by and if you have several hours like that then the days usually fly by as well.

There needs to be open constant communication between the therapist and front desk staff. Typically the front desk staff schedules the patients for the clinic while the therapists treat the patients when they are on their schedule. Ignorance of scheduling conflicts, problems, and productivity issues is no excuse and should never be accepted. The schedule is your lifeline in PT and needs to be managed effectively and efficiently. Patient cancels and reschedules are inevitable and need to be managed to prevent them from getting out of hand. You always want to reschedule versus cancel a patient. Rescheduling a patient can be done in the same day or the same week. If the patient calls to cancel, do not just say ok and hang up. Try to get a reason why they are canceling and offer them to reschedule to a later time that same day or another day that week. Also when a patient calls to cancel, that is a good time to verify that they will attend their next appointments and that they are scheduled. A lot of patients will cancel and not have another appointment scheduled, that is a great way for a patient to become forgotten about and never come back. That must be avoided at all costs and prevented when you establish communication with the patient.

Inactive patients are people that have not been seen for over a week in our system. If a patient has not been seen for over a week and we have not had communication with them over that time, then we call them to touch base and see why they have not been in therapy. Calling inactive patients is a thing all therapists must do to try and recover non-compliant patients and stay busy. Patients become inactive for many reasons but it is the job of the therapist and front desk staff to prevent them from becoming inactive and non-compliant.

No matter how many patients you call and try to reschedule and recover, some will not want to come to PT. Times are tough and money is tight in most households. For the most part PT is an elective purchase and the way the insurance companies are changing for the worse, PT is getting more expensive for patients. A common reason why people will not return to PT is due to a high co-payment, co-insurance, or deductible. I like to ask a patient during their initial evaluation what their thoughts are for PT visits. I'd rather see a patient 1 to 2 times a week for a couple weeks rather than only for the initial evaluation. You have to sell PT and that you are cutting them a break with only coming once a week, giving them a home exercise program, and that the doctor wants them to try some PT for a couple visits. The patient should feel like you are there to help them and coming 1-2 times a week versus 2-3 times a week is ok to do as long as they do the home exercise program that you give them and come a couple times a week.

One of the biggest problems in an outpatient orthopedic setting is how busy or slow a clinic and its staff are. Many clinics have several staff physical therapists that treat patients and that means having enough patients to fill everyone's schedule. When you are busy and the schedule is full, most of the time that is all you can ask for but being busy can cause conflict among your staff. Some staff could feel like they only want to treat one patient an hour while others want to see 2-3 patients an hour. That is why a productivity standard must be established and upheld for all staff. Regardless if a therapist wants to see more or less than the standard, the standard is set. Some will have higher productivity and some will have lower productivity but everyone should know the standard and accept it. The productivity standard is maintained by the schedule and is a great way to show how a therapist is doing and if they deserve a raise or not.

Chapter 21

Time Management

Physical therapy is all about time management. Proper time management is essential to make a good therapist into a great therapist. Achieving a high standard of time management and productivity should be a goal of all therapists. Time management is a trait that people can improve, but are most likely born with or have engrained in their personality. If you have it engrained in your personality or not, time management must be a trait of all therapists in order to treat patients, document properly, and provide quality care and interventions without lacking in one or any of those areas. Some therapists can document well but struggle with seeing more than one patient an hour or can see a lot of patients an hour and struggle to document well. To be a great therapist, you have to provide quality PT care to a lot of patients, document to a high standard without lacking information, and get everything done in a timely manner.

There are thousands of therapists in the world and they all have different motivations in life and with their career as a physical therapist. The standards of patient care, productivity, and documentation need to be established in your clinic and with yourself. By setting a standard, there will be expectations that all therapists need to uphold. It is tough to have a standard for time management, but time management will play a big part in achieving the standards for patient care, documentation, and productivity. If someone demonstrates proper time management then they most likely will be able to treat a lot of patients an hour, be able to document their daily notes well within that hour, and perform other daily tasks that may need to be completed (e.g. chart audits, cleaning, faxing documents, answering the phone).

The best way to think about time management is to divide each task you have to do and how much time you have to do it. Most therapists work 8-10 hour shifts 4-5 days a week and see around 12- 15 patients a day. Within those working hours, the physical therapist needs to perform patient care, properly document, keep the PT clinic nice, neat, and clean along with other miscellaneous tasks such as faxing notes to doctors, answering the phone, ordering supplies, and doing laundry. If you are not careful, patient care can eat up your whole day without completing your daily documentation notes. That last thing a physical therapist wants to do at the end of a long, tough, patient filled day is to complete 10-12 notes. It is best if you can complete your notes while the patient is still in the clinic and before you move on to treat another patient. It is something all therapists need to work on but after months and years of experience; you will develop your own way to manage all your daily tasks in a time efficient productive manner.

I find it best to multi-task with a combination of patient care and documentation within the same hour. For example, I try to start a daily note on my computer before I get the patient from the waiting room. I open the note and see what exercises they did last visit and develop a plan for the daily treatment. I walk up front to get the patient from the waiting room and escort them back to our PT gym. I ask questions about their condition and how they felt after last treatment. If possible, I start them on a bike, treadmill, arm bike, or pulleys. Once they are safely on a machine, I get subjective information from the patient about the area that we are treating. I ask about their condition, the pain, their functional mobility, strength, and performance of ADLs. I know they are safe on the equipment that I left them on (the bike, arm bike, pulleys, treadmill) so I go to my computer and complete my subjective and plan sections for the daily note I must complete for my patient. By starting the patient on exercises and knocking out two of the four sections for my daily SOAP note before the patient has completed their first exercise, puts me ahead of the game. With our computerized documentation, the objective section carries over from the previous note. Most of the time I do not have to add or change things to the objective section unless I am performing a re-evaluation or updating measurements on a patient. The only section left of my daily SOAP note is the assessment. The assessment must be done at the end of the patient treatment session as you cannot perform that section until you assess how they did with their exercises and are doing in general as a result of PT. It is a great idea to perform as much of your documentation that you can while your patients are safely performing exercises and do not require your immediate attention.

We time most of our exercises with actual timers in our clinic. Most exercises are performed between 2-3 minutes with the exception of the bike, modalities, and manual therapy which can usually be around 10 minutes for each intervention. If you put someone on the bike for 10 minutes, you have a free 10 minutes to start your notes, treat another patient, or do another task. Freeing up 10 minutes of your time between patients or notes is much desired. A free 10 minutes is a lot of time to complete a lot of things. I try to get my notes started early and completed within the same hour that my patients are in the clinic and that can only be done by freeing up a couple minutes throughout the treatment hour. If you wait to complete your notes, then the notes usually may be missing some information or be incomplete with what actually occurred that treatment session. There is too much room for error if you wait to the end of the day to complete 10-12 notes. My goal with documentation is to complete the notes within the same hour that the patient is treated and have the noted signed by the therapist as the patient is leaving the clinic. That simple method is one that I try to complete with every patient that I treat. It is much easier said than done but needs to be the standard for yourself and your clinic. If you set your standards high than you will be achieving success without trying and your success will come with your normal daily effort.

Simply put, time management is about managing your time. When I think time management, I think it is all about doing the most that you can within the least amount of time. Physical therapy is about treating patients hour to hour and how much you can complete within that hour. The tasks within each hour will vary, so proper time management is important in order to maintain high efficiency and productivity. When treating more than one patient an hour, proper time management must be utilized to provide quality PT care along with proper documentation for each patient. Teaching your patients several exercises and developing a patient routine of exercises will save you time, stress, and frustration when treating more than one patient an hour. When a patient arrives early, if possible, try to start them early especially if you are double or tripled booked for the hour. Gaining a free 10-15 minutes goes a long way when you have 2-3 patients under your care during the same hour. You need to find little tricks to free up a couple minutes here and there, so you can devote equal attention to you patients or other tasks that need to be done during the same time as patient care. In PT, therapists live hour to hour and one hour to the next can be drastically different. One hour you might be seeing one patient an hour and the next you may be treating three patients in the same hour. Treating more than one patient an hour is not always as bad as it sounds and it can actually be fun and productive if managed correctly and efficiently with proper time management standards and principles.

Chapter 22

Referrals from Doctors

A physical therapist is only as good as the patients they treat and make better. If you do not get any patients from doctors, then you cannot have a successful career as a physical therapist. It is a simple statement but one that a lot of therapist do not think about. Doctors and really the front desk staff of a doctor's office are the gatekeepers to how busy or slow a PT clinic will be. The way the medical model is setup in the United States is that a patient must see a medical doctor (MD) first before coming to physical therapy. For the most part that is a good thing, more medical opinions the better when treating patients. That is great when a MD actually refers his patients to a center that he does not own or have a financial part in. There is great debate if PT offices that are physician owned practices (POPs) should even be allowed to exist, but that debate is for another book.

To be successful as a physical therapist you need to treat patients and a lot of them. Physical therapy is a numbers game, how many patients can you see in one hour, in one day and one month? The only way to get patients is for a patient to be referred to your practice by a MD, so hopefully you will see a benefit to getting to know some local doctors around your physical therapy practice. The more a doctor trusts your abilities as a therapist the more patients he will usually send your way. The best way for a MD to trust your abilities is to see how you handle one of his patients, so getting to know the local doctors is a must.

You have to get a meet and greet or a lunch with a doctor and his office staff so you can see what kind of doctor they are. Are they a conservative doctor, aggressive MD, does the doctor have protocols, all great questions that you have to find out by meeting them. There is no way around it; you have to make the local referring physicians remember how great of a PT you really are. All you need is a couple of good patients that report back to the MD and thank him for sending them to you. But first you have to get the MD to refer to you and then to keep them sending you patients based on patient compliments and reports back to the MD.

Now all the being said, you can bust you butt have lunches with the doctor and staff, shadow them during their office hours, observe surgeries and still not get any patients from them. Marketing with MDs is only good if you get business from them and sometimes you need to be direct and ask for a couple patients to build that trust up and form the doctor PT relationship. Please do not get discouraged when MDs do not refer to your office, be persistent, ask for the business, and continue to build honest trustworthy relationships.

Referrals from doctors should be one of the biggest focuses of marketing and how to grow your business. Without referrals from doctor's offices you most likely will not be able to survive in the PT business. Building, maintaining, and growing business relationships with doctors and the doctor's office staff are essential to maintain a busy schedule and treat a lot of patients. Doctors want to know that will treat their patient safely, effectively, and efficiently. All doctors want to feel that you are working just for them, that you get their patients in when the patients want to come in, and that you are there to serve the doctor and only them. Of course you do not only treat one doctor's patients but you want to make the doctor feel that you go above and beyond only for him and his patients.

After you setup a professional relationship with a doctor's office, you must keep that relationship strong and current. By calling, sending progress notes and re-evaluations, and having regular communication with the doctor and his staff you can keep a good quality referral connection strong for years. A good referring doctor can be a blessing and a curse at the same time however. Many doctors office trust a PT and his staff after several positive patient experiences but it is important to make the doctor's office love sending you patients and working with you. Even if that means you have to bend over backwards and work harder for a doctor's office and their patients. Some doctor's offices send patients with multiple body parts to treat and that requires more effort and work for the therapists. It will be frustrating at times but keeping a good referral source happy is the name of the game and must be done. Once a doctor and his staff become unhappy with a PT and a clinic they will not refer any patients to that office. Remember that when treating a patient and if a problem with a patient is worth losing a referral source over.

Chapter 23

How to Grow Your PT Business

The formula to be successful in any field let alone the medical field is you need customers to buy your service or product. The best way to be successful in PT is to treat a lot of patients and get them better. The best way to grow your business is to make people want to come back to you and your clinic for every injury, ache and pain, and dysfunction. Making patients love coming to see you so much that they will refer their loved ones and friends to your services because they enjoyed your treatment so much should be a goal of every PT and PT business.

You can be the best PT but if doctors and patients do not know you exist, then what good are you? Healthcare is all about relationships and referrals to different disciplines. Medical doctors (MD) and orthopedic surgeons are two main people that you need to target to help grow your therapist case load, productivity, and business. A good referral source such as an orthopedic surgeon can refer hundreds of patients to your clinic each year.

Another great way to grow your business besides marketing yourself to local doctors is to increase your education and certifications. Some doctors will only send their patients to therapists with certain certifications such as orthopedic certified specialist (OCS) and manual therapy certification (MTC). So by increasing your education and knowledge in certain areas, local doctors will trust in your abilities as a therapist that you are educated in ways to get their patients better.

To be successful and grow your PT business, you must focus on 3 areas for proper short term and long term growth. First and most important you need to market and meet with the local referral sources around your clinic. Second, once you get a lot of patients you need to keep them coming back and telling their referring doctors that they loved working with you and they would recommend using you again. Doctors love taking credit for sending their patient to good PT clinics and taking the recognition for your efforts and knowledge. Of course you cannot and most likely will not be able to make every patient extremely happy with their PT treatment but you need to try and accommodate almost every patient request and idea unless it is unsafe or not recommended for the patient. Thirdly and most importantly, you need to manage your costs, budget, productivity, utilities, hours, and schedule.

A PT clinic will not grow let alone survive if it does not have patients to treat and profit from. You need to constantly be evaluating the needs of the clinic, the best hours for patient care and scheduling, and the costs to run the clinic every day, week, and month. No matter what state or practice you are in, insurances will only pay so much for PT sessions, so you need to know how to manage the different insurance reimbursement rates and the best way to maximize your revenue. One of the biggest payers for PT is Medicare. Medicare can be a great payer if you manage them correctly such as getting 4 units of time based service, never grouping patients together, and correctly billing your treatment times for each charge category such as therapeutic exercise, therapeutic activities, and so forth.

Times are tough in the world and people do not have a lot of extra income for purchases or services that are elective such as physical therapy. For the most part, PT is not needed to save a patient's life and so most people do not want to come to PT any longer then they have to. I cannot count how many times a patient is a onetime visit for their initial evaluation and refuses to come back due to a high insurance co-payment and general financial issues. It is better to have a patient come once a week for a couple weeks instead of coming for only one visit and never come back.

You might have to sell PT and how it will benefit the patient by coming back for another visit or two. Remember that you cannot get someone better if they do not come in for treatment so it is important to communicate about how PT will make them better and what your plan is for them over the next PT visits.

"When do I see you again?" That question is an easy line that must be asked at the end of each patient treatment by every therapist to every patient that they see. That single simple question opens the lines of communication of when they are coming back and verification of what time and day. When that question is not asked, patients say their good byes and might just walk out the clinic without scheduling or knowing when they have another appointment with you. If that question is asked then you can make sure they are scheduled for another appointment and there is no excuse to why the patient is not seen again. Communication is a must to have with your patients to ensure patient compliance with PT treatments, visits, and home exercise programs. Growth of your business can be as simple as that you are seeing your patients for more visits and that question is a great way to communicate compliance of PT scheduled visits.

Patients will be non-compliant with PT visits for various reasons and a great way to grow your business is to recover patients that have not been seen for several weeks. Workers compensation patients can be very trying patients for many reasons but a common one is due to non-compliance. A great way to make a patient become more compliant with PT is to make it known that the patient will be discharged from PT if they miss too many scheduled PT sessions. If that does not work then a discharge should be sent to the MD and workers compensation case manager. Sometimes the MD and case manager might not be aware that the patient has been missing appointments or not even scheduling return visits. By opening the lines of communication you can get the

MD and case manager on your side and have the pressure put on the patient to resume PT care. Most of the time just by doing a simple discharge summary and faxing it to the MD and case manager, the patient will be sent back to PT and resume PT care due to a fear of losing their workers compensation injury claim. The discharge summary is a great way to communicate with the MD and case managers that you tried to get the patient better but due to patient self-discharge or non-compliance you can no longer continue care. Most MDs and case manager will not accept a patient being non-compliant with PT and will push the patient to come back to your clinic.

Chapter 24

"Be Like a Chameleon"

I use this phrase to make PT students and fellow PTs understand that you need to treat each patient that you see differently and accordingly to their needs, personalities, and functional deficits. You need to adapt to your patients and environment just like a chameleon blends into their environment to maximize their safety and well-being. All patients are not created equal, even patients with similar pathologies or injuries of the same body part can vary how they are treated in PT. You need to adapt to all patients and change your plan of care accordingly to fully maximize each patients rehab potential.

In PT you will treat many different types of patient from different backgrounds, ages, states, and functional levels. In a typical day as a PT in the outpatient orthopedic setting I see about 18+ patients in an 11 hour day that range from young teenage athletic injuries to the elderly dealing with arthritis in most of their body. When giving patients exercises and education you need to develop a way to educate each individual patient the best way so they understand what needs to be done to make them better.

We see a wide array of patients in outpatient orthopedics every day. One hour you are treating an elderly man and his arthritic lumbar spine, the next you are seeing a teenage soccer player for a hip flexion strain, and you end your day treating a former military person for a rotator cuff problem. With all those patients you need to maintain interest, focus, and fun even if they are not the most exciting patient. I know myself I learn a lot from my patients and take a genuine interest in how they are doing while in PT and outside of my care. I keep treatment fun, exciting, but direct and specific to getting them better. That is much easier said than done but after years of experience in your setting and clinic, you will develop your style of fun, excitement, and functional based treatment.

One of the worst things you can do as a PT or PT student is to not be able to relate to your patients and make them feel comfortable with being in therapy. Please, if you are a student never say to a patient," Well I'm sorry but we have not learned that in school yet so I cannot help you." That will almost certainly make the patient never want to work with you again and trust that you know what you are doing. We had a student say that to a patient when they were asked about the lumbar spine and their condition. If you do not know something, then say something such as, "I am not sure but I will look into that for you" or "Well every patient is a little different so it could take a little longer for your situation." Sometimes generic answers are what you need to give when you are not sure about something. Patients want to trust in your knowledge and abilities. When that trust is gone, it is almost impossible to get it back, so please do not do anything to lose it in the first place.

Being able to listen and have a conversation with a patient all while making sure they are doing their exercises and maximizing their rehab potential is a key to quality patient care. Some of your patients will talk your ear off, while others will barely say anything. That is where being like a chameleon is key, you need to bring a patient out of their shell and feel comfortable with talking and having fun in PT or tone it down and have a patient focus more on exercises and treatment rather than talking and being too social. There is no problem with being social with patients but they are not in PT for a social gathering. Patients need to work and be social at the same time. Maintaining patient focus while having fun and be talkative may be tough for some patients but it must be done and achieved through a blending of the two areas.

Chapter 25

Certifications & Continuing Education Units

To be one of the best physical therapists you can possibly be, you need to stay up on the latest evidence based practice and techniques. The best way to stay up on proper treatment and the latest evidence based medicine is to attend continuing education (CE) courses on subjects that will benefit your treatment of patients in your clinic. For example I work in an outpatient clinic and see a lot of backs, shoulders, and knee pathologies so naturally the best courses for me are treatments based on the back, shoulder and knees.

Every two years you are required to complete 24 Continuing Education Hours (CEUs) which will need to consist of 2 hours of medical errors training and 22 hours of state certified PT hours. If you are a new grad then you will need to earn 2 hours in AIDS/HIV education but only in your first renewal period of 2 years after you are initially licensed. There are various websites that will cover the medical errors (www.cheapceus.com) part of your CEU requirements. The remaining 22 hours needs to be done through weekend courses, conferences, certification programs, or online CEUs courses. Make sure when taking a course that it is eligible for CEUs in your state, not all courses are eligible in every state, especially if you travel out of the state for a course.

Some of the very best physical therapists have more than one certification alongside their PT credentials. I myself have CSCS and COMT along with my DPT. I recommend getting as much education as possible especially if your company will pay for it. The American Physical Therapy Association (APTA) has several great certification programs for each area of interest of PT. I myself will most likely be taking the orthopedic certification specialist (OCS) or sports certification specialist (SCS) as I will benefit from that material in my outpatient sports setting. If you are interested another specialty, check the website www.apta.org and see if they have a certification program that you may be interested in.

The fact of the matter is that people want to see therapists that are smart, educated, interesting, and can get them better. Doctors want to send their patients to reliable, qualified, and knowledgeable therapists that have certifications and specialties that show education and training. The more education, training, and qualifications you have, the more likely a doctor with trust his patients with your care. Not all courses, programs, and certifications are created equal but are beneficial for continued education, growth, and knowledge. I urge all therapists whether they are new grads or a veteran that has been a therapist for many years to take courses on material that interest them and/or will benefit their clinics. CEU courses are not the end all be all of PT so you need to make the executive decision about what is taught and how you will carry that over to your daily practice with patients. Course instructors teach material that they are knowledgeable about, but that does not mean that everything that they teach should be done on all your patients. Hopefully they will teach you techniques and education and really push the idea of taking the knowledge from the course into your clinics with an open mind but knowing that you cannot and should not try everything they teach you on every patient that you see.

Obtaining more certifications and credentials will not usually increase your salary based on the credentials but those extra certifications will allow for better jobs and positions. Doctors will send more patients to you based on your credentials which in turn will bring more revenue to the clinic and hopefully more money to you. More education and credentials will ensure job security and make you an asset to the company and in your PT clinic.

Chapter 26

How to Perform a Great Functional Evaluation

Great care of patients always starts with the initial evaluation and mainly the subjective and objective parts of their examination. You gain so much knowledge about the patient and their condition by just asking some questions and performing some tests on the patient. By asking, "How did this happen?" you may find out the mechanism of injury, or by asking, "When does your pain or problem bother you?" you may be able to tell what type of tissue is involved. A lot of times a patient will describe their pain, conditions, or symptoms and you will get more information from that then a diagnosis or prescription from a doctor. Sometimes a prescription that a patient brings from the doctor's office them tells you basic information about the injury and/or surgery. For example, a patient might come in with a prescription from a doctor that just says shoulder pain or even just left shoulder. You then need to ask the patient what is going on with their shoulder, when does it hurt, what makes it better/worse, and start your evaluation with a question and answer part to try to find what is going on with their pathology and how PT will help.

A common sense approach to PT is what you need most of the time and especially when performing an initial evaluation of a patient. You can poke and provoke pain in most patients very easily, but they are not coming there for you make them worse of course. Patients want your help to improve or even get rid of the pain/sx altogether. For every patient you need to perform ROM, MMT, special tests, functional tests, and anything else to find out what is going on with the patient. Please pick and choose appropriate tests and measures for each individual patient. Do not have a patient perform a squat test or single leg balance test if they cannot rise out of the chair without pain or difficulty or cannot stand with both feet on the ground without difficulty. I love the mindset of if you have to look too hard at something it probably is not that important. I carry that mindset over to my patients with examination and evaluation.

Range of motion (ROM) is the first objective measure I perform on a patient. No matter what body part you are treating, observing ROM is necessary for all patients. Functional levels of ROM are what are expected to gain while in PT and you have to know a patients baseline values for each motion and muscle action. Active ROM and Passive ROM must both be completed to tell if there is a contractile, non-contractile, or both types of tissue dysfunction. By simply asking a patient to perform ROM in different motions you can tell quality of motion, functional level of motion, and manual muscle test grade. A 3/5 manual muscle test grade is when a patient can perform full ROM against gravity without resistance. If a patient does not have full ROM with a specific movement then they cannot have a grade of 3/5 or greater. If someone does not have at least full ROM then I most likely will not even manually resist their movement, as they cannot have any higher than a 3-/5 MMT. Based on how much ROM a person has I will grade the MMT accordingly. Such as if a patient had 90 degrees of the normal 180 degrees of motion then they will get a grade of 2-/5 or 2/5 for that motion.

Manual Muscle Testing (MMT) is not very functional at all, it needs to be done but I don't find too much strength in knowing if someone is a 4/5 or 4+/5 with shoulder flexion. I'd rather see them perform a functional reach, or carry, or perform an action that causes pain or is difficult to perform. You can gain so much more by evaluating posture, functional task ability, and specific muscle actions. That being said, if a patient has a low MMT grade such as 3-

/5 or even 2/5 then we know that the patient has a functional deficit that needs to be treated and improved.

I love to perform functional objective measures for all patients when they are appropriate. Unless the patient is status post-surgery and cannot perform a test due to restriction of stressing healing tissue and safety, I have my patients perform tasks that they will most likely perform every day. The most functional test I perform for the upper extremity and cervical spine is the Apley's functional scratch test. Functional reach testing is important as it will show quality of movement to complete ADLs and basic care that everyone must do every day. For example a person has to comb their hair, get dressed, and reach for things. The functional testing will show how your patients perform those tasks and the results of your functional testing will make it easier for you to develop a plan of care and treatment goals. The most functional test I perform for the lower extremity is the squat and lateral step down tests. Squats and lateral step downs are great exercises to evaluate knee pain, genu valgum, and overall leg strength. Both tests will be useful in seeing quality of movement and functional aspects that every patient will do every day.

The purpose of the initial evaluation is to develop a plan of care for treatment of impairments, dysfunctions, muscular imbalances, and symptoms that the patient is complaining of. That being said, of course you need to detect the cause of the problems and then see if you can treat them in physical therapy. The initial evaluation should be done as efficiently, effectively, and safely as possible. In one hour with a patient you should have uncovered a great amount of subjective information, performed several functional objective measures, developed a plan of care if treatment is medically necessary, and performed some treatment on the patient. That might seem like a lot do in an hour but you can group objective measures and treatment in the same activity to save time and ask some subjective questions while performing objective measures. Killing two birds with one stone as often as possible will help your time management while performing an initial evaluation especially if the patient is late to their appointment and you might have to work a little faster with the patient due to time constraints.

There is no magic way to perform an evaluation due to the simple fact that not all patients will be able to tolerate everything that you do. Not all low back patients will be able to tolerate every special test or will present with the need to perform the same special tests. A great way to perform evaluation is with a general plan in mind and be able to adjust your plan on the fly for each specific patient. For example if you have a patient that is diagnosed with left shoulder pain, don't laugh that is a real diagnosis that we get from doctors, what would be your first thing to focus on? I would think to get a thorough history about what happened to start making the shoulder hurt, what makes it better/worse, how does it limit you, is it getting better since it starting bothering you and finally did you get any imaging done like a MRI or X-ray? Based on the answers that were provided by the patient, I could get an idea of what objective measures to perform. The objective measure section is where therapists will differ on what is important and not important to focus on during an evaluation. The best objective measures in my mind are functionally based and important for provocation of symptoms that the patient is suffering from. For all patients you must have a basis of ROM, strength, joint mobility, functional movements, posture, palpation, DTR, dermatomes and myotomes for the involved and uninvolved sides of the body.

It is easy to think of an initial evaluation as a time that you should only perform manual muscle testing (MMT), active and passive ROM, joint mobility, special tests, and palpation. They are all great tools and should be done during an evaluation but with time and experience you should be to perform all those techniques in about 10 to 15 minutes with proper form, technique, and diagnostic ability. If something is not obvious or stands out to me I move on to some other measure or test to try to reproduce the patient's pain and symptoms they are experiencing outside of PT. You will get a lot of patients that are limited with ROM, strength, flexibility, mobility; show poor posture, and have functional limitations. Those patients are easy to treat and easy to diagnose due to the obvious impairments and dysfunctions that you found. For the patients that do not show obvious impairments and treatable dysfunctions, then you must observe functional movements and tasks such as squatting, gait, transfers, bridging, and going up and down steps. Functional tasks will display a lot of objective measurable information that will help you design an appropriate plan of care.

In summary, anything and everything you do during an evaluation should have a purpose. If there is no reason why you are having them do an exercise, test, measure or activity then you probably should not be doing it. An efficient evaluation should be done within 30 minutes on average. Of course you will have some outliers where it takes you 45 or even 60 minutes to perform a thorough evaluation and develop a plan of care. In my book functional tasks such as transfers, squatting, steps, and balance will usually show more impairments dysfunctions than your traditional PT school diagnostic measures. The best clinician will perform the standard objective measures such as MMTs, ROM, and palpation along with the addition of more on relevant functional tasks and activities.

Chapter 27

PT Treatment Interventions

Patients come to physical therapy to get better, improve their function, and increase their strength and general well-being. Now that can be achieved by different methods of treatment, education, and information. Some patients will not improve as much as they would like no matter how much treatment they receive. Others will getter better pretty quickly and achieve quick results and good outcomes. There are so many different interventions, treatments, and modalities that a therapist can perform but every patient will respond differently to treatment, so the therapist needs to adapt and develop a specific plan for each specific patient.

Physical therapy treatment can and should consist of several different methods and practices. The best outcomes are usually achieved with a combination of treatments, such as therapeutic exercise, self-care home management, manual therapy, neuromuscular re-education, patient education, modalities, and a patient specific home exercise program. Through some sort of combination of those interventions that is specific to the patients' needs, impairments, and imbalances the patient should improve and increase their function. Many research articles show that the best outcomes are achieved with a combination of exercise and manual therapy. I like to add the aspect of education and a home exercise program into the mix because people are definitely outside of PT more than they are in PT. You can do the best 1 hour long treatment 2-3x a week with the patient leaving the clinic feeling great only to undo everything you just did and exacerbate their pain and symptoms with poor practices at home. That has happened to me and will happen to you unless you achieve proper patient compliance and teach them about our team of two approach strategy.

Therapeutic exercise is the number one billed code in all of PT. So many treatment exercises are classified as therapeutic exercise. With thousands of different exercises classified as therapeutic exercise you can see that it is easy to bill most treatments under that category. Every patient that comes to PT should do some sort of therapeutic exercise in their daily treatments. That being said, you need to think of therapeutic exercise as your staple of treatments and develop different ways to train and strengthen a muscle. Straight leg raises, heel raises, recumbent bike, leg press, and many others are considered therapeutic exercise. Basic exercise is boring to the patient and needs to be spiced up, enhanced, and improved after a couple of visits. There are many different ways to achieve proper muscle contraction, kinematics and motion and your patients will want to mix it up after a couple of sessions. The best way to do that is to create a list in your mind or even on paper of how to a perform exercises to work each and every muscle in the body and how to advance or change the aspect of the exercise to improve overload, recruitment, and general strengthening. Basic exercises like straight leg raises, isometrics, and heel raises can and should be put in a patients home exercise program and only done at home after they show proper exercise technique, compliance, and form.

Some of the best therapists have been educated and taught hundreds or even thousands of exercises and exercise progressions that they use on a daily basis for all of their patients. Therapeutic exercises are a key component in physical therapy and therapists need to know how to properly perform them, progress them, and alter them. Patients will be coming in for a variety of impairments, dysfunctions, and symptoms. As a therapist you need to know or how to figure out a proper plan of care that will usually consist of many different interventions, exercises, education, and modalities. Exercises need to become second nature to a therapist. When a patient comes in for knee or shoulder pain, a proficient therapist will be able to automatically think of a bunch of exercises to work the muscles and surrounding area of the injury, impairment, or dysfunction. If someone comes in for knee pain, you should be thinking of exercises that the patient might be able to do and by process of elimination based on the objective measures that you found during the evaluation, daily treatment, and re-evaluations. If the patient demonstrates quad weakness after injury then you should think of how to make the quad stronger by doing the proper concentric and eccentric muscle functions. The quadriceps muscles perform knee extension and hip flexion, so you should think about having the patient do every exercise to perform those actions. For example, to work the quads I would have the patient do the bike, leg press, leg extension, lateral step down, steps forward and lateral, squats, straight legs raises, hip flexion, Swiss ball knee rolls, hip adductor isometric ball squeezes and bridging. Maybe the patient can perform some of those exercises, all of them, or modified versions of those exercises. The exercises are one aspect of a patient's treatment but the 1 hour long treatment will flow much better if you have a plan in your head with what exercises to do with the patient and can move from exercise to exercise without missing a beat.

Patients like to know that their therapist knows what they are doing and moving from one exercise to the next with no hesitation or problem shows that you are confident with the exercise choices and are competent as a therapist. That is where having a mental exercise sheet in your head comes in handy. Patients do not like it when therapists are unsure of themselves or not sure if the patient should be doing an exercise. Communication on why a patient is doing an exercise and what they are working is a great way for patients to understand what the plan is in PT and that their therapist is competent at their job.

Therapeutic exercise is the number one billed code in PT but that is not the only billable code that we have. Manual therapy, therapeutic activities, neuromuscular re-education, gait training, and self-care/home management are the other staples of CPT billing codes. When a therapist puts their hands on a patient for ROM, joint mobility, soft tissue techniques, or providing manual resistance than that will fall under manual therapy. Therapeutic activities will fall under anything that a person does under normal activity such as lifting, pulling, reaching, and any other job demand functions. Now that sounds like therapeutic exercise but the activity can be done with a box or other job related items. Neuromuscular re-education is mostly used for patients who had surgery and require those techniques to have the muscles to fire correctly again. For example when a patient had ACL surgery and their quad needs to relearn to fire again, then a quad set will be billed under neuromuscular re-education for that specific patient. Gait training is what we use for patients when we are working on the gait pattern and specific gait kinematics of the gait cycle. Gait is our fancy word for walking but gait training is our billed code for when skilled techniques are used to improve the patients proper gait cycle. Self-care/home management is a forgotten billed code but a very important one. Anytime you teach a patient about a home exercise program, proper posture, using ice at home, or anything else to help treat their pain/symptoms and dysfunction then you will most likely bill that education under that code. The self-care/home management code is underutilized to say the least and needs to be a staple of your treatment billable codes. Giving someone information and education about their condition and how to make them better is valuable and skilled which should equal billable and revenue generating.

Chapter 28

State Practice Acts

An important area that most PT students and licensed therapists do not think about when it comes to treatment and patient care is what can and cannot be done in regards to their state practice acts. State practice acts are what will limit therapists to what they can and cannot do. In the state of Florida we cannot do a couple different treatments that I know you can do in other states. In Florida, you are not allowed to puncture the skin for any reason. Some treatment such as dry needling is not allowed to be performed by a PT along with suture and staple removal since you have to puncture the skin to remove the material. It might not seem like a big deal but those are just two examples of how your state practice act can and will limit your abilities as a therapist.

Knowing your state practice act is very important especially if you are a therapist that moved into a new state to practice PT. Practicing in one state does not carryover to another state. If you are practicing as a licensed PT in a state you must obey the state practice acts or can face penalties or even loss of your PT license. Finding out what your state practice act consists of can be done easily online through the APTA website (http://www.apta.org/Licensure/StatePracticeActs/).

When in doubt check the state practice acts to be safe and to know if you can or cannot provide an intervention. Ignorance of the state practice act is not an acceptable excuse and will not provide any relief if actions are brought against a therapist. Practice acts must be upheld by all costs and there are no exceptions. Please research of what you can and cannot do as a PT if you are unsure even the slightest bit. It is better to be safe than sorry.

Chapter 29

Management

Every clinic, hospital, SNF and really any location that has physical therapy has a manager of the facility and staff. Most people like to think that they can be a manager and that it is easy. For some PT clinics that might be true but for the majority of them it is not an easy job. I myself became a center manager somewhat early in my career due to a great opportunity becoming available to me. I worked as a staff PT for a year in a half before becoming a manager. My situation and experience is definitely the exception to rule and nowhere close to the norm. Most people have to work years before a management job opens up. If a manager job opens up and you are up to the challenge, then try it out and see if being a manager is right for you.

I believe a great manager works hard, leads by example, and practices what he preaches. I know myself if a manager did not do the three things listed above, I would not respect him as much as I should or would if he showed me those 3 attributes. Upper management does not get a lot of respect with staff therapists and people I call "in the trenches" from day to day. We all know a person who works for a company where their boss or upper management keep making decisions that make no sense and cause extra work/stress for their workers with day to day tasks. Policies made by management should be made to improve the company along with the well-being of its employees. In a perfect world, policies would be made to help everyone but as we all know that is definitely not the case.

It is easy to manage great employees and yourself when you have an enjoyable work environment, great employees who share the same views and goals of the job, and a busy productive schedule. On the other hand, you can only make an employee do so much that they do not want to do, be so busy, and treat so many patients. My advice for all managers is to be able to hire your staff from the beginning, starting with your front desk person. They are the front lines of your clinic; they schedule patients, verify insurances, submit billing, and do a lot of tasks to make the clinic run smoothly. Next you have to have great staff therapists that will perform the bulk of your evaluations, treatments, and generate revenue through patient care. I manage a part time physical therapist assistant (PTA), a physical therapist (PT), an occupational therapist (OT), and a front desk person along with myself. We do not have a huge clinic with a huge staff but enough to make good revenue for the company and not be too crazy with problems.

Center managers of PT clinics do much more than just sit around and supervise their employees. At least a good one does. To be a good manager you need to be well rounded in all aspects of patient care, employee management, problem solving, and the business financials. I like to be available to my employees and make them feel that they can come to me with problems, questions, or help with patient care, billing, and general inquiries but stay far enough away so that I am not considered a micro manager. Providing help when necessary but giving therapists the freedom to provide care their individual way as long as it is safe, effective, and the patients enjoy coming to therapy. Problems will arise in every occupation and you need effective managers to help solve them when they spring up and prevent them from happening when possible. That sounds like common sense but not every person is capable of making tough decisions and having hard conversations with employees about poor performance or disciplinary actions. One of the hardest situations of being a center manager is not being able to provide an employee with something that they want. Whether it is an annual raise, time off that they requested, or even the ability to come in or leave early. I am a firm believer of helping those that help you but in certain situations you might not always be able to accommodate therapist requests.

Business and mainly the finances of your PT clinic will ultimately show how successful you and your clinic are. "You are only as good as your numbers are" is a great phrase that shows how upper management and business people think. In therapy we are treating people and the human body, we are not selling hamburgers. People will cancel, be non-compliant, and generally give you the run around with visits and treatment. "How can I help it if my patients will not come in for therapy?" is a great question I hear a lot from therapists that are having cancellations and holes in their schedules. The easy answer to that question is nothing, but there are simple things that can be done to prevent a patient from cancelling a lot or becoming non-compliant with visits. Now they will not work for all patients and they will not stop patients that cancel due to sickness, personal conflicts, or doctor appointments but may work for a patient who might cancel due to lack of interest or high co-pays. We can usually prevent a patient from cancelling with some easy simple communication skills and increase our overall schedule productivity, revenue, and business in the clinic. The name of the game is all about getting your patients in and keeping them coming back to PT. Usually we try to get our patients that are non-surgical patients treated for 8-10 visits then discharge to a home program. If the patient had surgery then that will vary on the degree and amount of tissue repaired but most likely around 3 to 4 months of PT is needed.

"Fair but firm" is a slogan that I love to refer to with management. It means that there are standards and expectations for every job but they are fair in achieving them. PT is no different and is a great career for that slogan. You need to have fair achievable productivity standards that everyone is aware of. If everyone knows the rules of the game then they can achieve success and win. If your staff does not meet the standards and expectations then they should not be expecting bonuses, raises, and other incentive based rewards. Being fair with your employees shows that you care about them and their abilities at work. Being firm at the same time shows that you are tough and will uphold the standards without exception.

Going from a staff PT to a center manager is a great opportunity for anyone and I encourage everyone to go for it, if an opportunity arises. It can be a scary, pressure filled, nerve racking experience but worth it, if you have the right environment for growth and success. I was lucky enough to become a manager fairly early in the PT career and have seen and dealt with a lot of challenges. Being a center manager overall is great and a lot of fun but as the person in charge you are the one to blame and fix problems along with getting the benefits of a higher salary, bonuses, and more time off. I have only been a manager for a couple years now but have learned and will continue to learn valuable lessons from my experiences and problems that arise. Almost everything that could go wrong did go wrong within my first year as a center manager but I made it through even when it was tough and I did not see a light at the end of the tunnel. If I could survive my first year of management with minimal bumps and scars, then anyone can.

Chapter 30

My First year of Management

As I wrote in the previous chapter, I have been a manager for a couple years now but remember my first year as a center manger like it was yesterday. I first became a staff PT for a major PT company in south Florida that is nationally run and has over 900 clinics in the United States. I worked in south Florida for a year and a half before moving to the Tampa Bay area to transfer to a clinic and become a center manager. I moved into a new area not knowing anyone in the area or at the clinic that I was going to be managing. The clinic that I took over had a full time PT, part time OT, and full time front desk person. I was the new guy on the block and felt an immediate sense that I was disrupting their way of life in the clinic and they did not like it. Ultimately I was sent there to turn the clinic around and make it successful as it was not hitting its monthly numbers, had poor productivity, and was barely making ends meet to turn a profit. If the clinic was successful or had proper management already then I would not have had the opportunity to accept the management position.

Being the new guy I did not want to rock the boat too much too quickly and tried to focus on building a connection with the clinic staff. After about two to three months, I saw several areas that needed to be improved to get the clinic running smoothly, efficiently, and to turn profitable. Knowing that the staff would not like the changes I wanted to implement, I needed to have a meeting and present the changes that were going to be started immediately. First, I had to make the staff work when they were supposed to work and be at the clinic. The staff would not come in until their first patient even if the clinic was open but no patient was scheduled. The clinic schedule had way too many holes in the schedule. Holes in the schedule are horrible for business, productivity, and profitability. So clearly the PT only wanted to work the bare basic schedule and get paid for full time 40 hours a week. The PT was a salaried employee so it made no difference to her if she treated 4 or 14 patients, as she would get paid the same. The front desk person could sit there all day with barely anything to do and get paid for being on the computer. As you can see the clinic staff had started being lazy, unproductive, and did not really care. Being the new center manager in training I had to turn the clinic around, increase productivity, and start making profit for the company.

After I made major changes with the schedule, made the staff be in the clinic even if you did not have a patient, and trying to keep our patients coming back to therapy, my staff and I started to have conflicts. I wanted the clinic to improve and be a great place for PT. The staff could care less and just wanted to see a couple patients a day and get a pay check. After several meetings and one big argument, my staff knew that I was for real and was not going anywhere. Sensing a new flow to the clinic and a new standard was established, my front desk person quit and my full time 40 hour PT decided to work 32 hours a week. So I lost 8 hours a week from a PT and had to hire a new front desk person. I was mad, uneasy, and unsure about the new changes and challenges that were presented to me within the first 3 months of working at the new clinic. Looking back now, that was a turning point to my success and growth. I felt that I was right in all aspects that needed to be changed for the growth and improvement of the clinic. I was easy going with most things but not about the schedule, productivity standard of 1.5 patients per hour, and how to make money for the clinic.

I easily could have went into the new clinic tried to be friends with everyone, look the other way with mistakes and problems that were occurring, and barely made any changes. That is not what I was hired to do and would not have been accepted by my boss. As a center manager you need to make tough unpopular decisions at times and if you cannot do that then management is not for you. Productivity, success, profit, and patient care are the only things that should matter at first glance and especially if you are a new manager. If previous staff and the way things were done prior to your arrival are getting in the way of success and growth, then major changes need to be done to be successful. Hiring, firing, and new roles for staff might need to be done so expect some changes, compromises, and tough tasks awaiting your new role as center manager. My boss knew I had a tough road ahead of me but knew that I could get the job done and made sure that I had his full support.

After about 7 to 8 months of quality leadership, management, and the hiring of new staff, we had turned the clinic around and were productive, profitable, and providing quality PT. I hired a new front desk person, setup better OT hours to maximize revenue and scheduling, and I was more involved with patient care and treatment. With help from my market manager we had a recipe for success and growth. To be successful in PT, you cannot do it alone and I know that firsthand. Even the best PT needs help with patient care, billing & coding, and scheduling. If you try to do it alone then you will have too much stress and become overwhelmed with too much on your plate.

Around the one year mark of being a center manager, I had to deal with a couple more hiccups in the road. My OT was going to be retiring at the end the year, so we had to interview and find a new OT for the job. If that was not bad enough my full time staff PT was going on maternity leave due to high risk pregnancy and needed to be on bed rest. I would be down to one therapist at the end of the year with no plan of how to make it work. We started looking for a new OT right away and I had to pick up the slack on the PT side. I treated 3-4 patients an hour pretty regularly for about 4 months until we got some help from a part time therapist. The staffing template took a hit but eventually we hired a new OT and transitioned a new PT between my center and another to help maximize productivity and patient care. It was a rough couple of months but we made it through and actually made a good profit and revenue with the adjusted schedules and therapist models.

My first year of management was a crazy, hectic, problematic, bumpy road that I am amazed that I survived from. I felt pressure from the job, from my boss, and my employees but managed to make everyone as happy as I could. Many lessons were learned that I still carry with me today and will in the future. You have to learn some lessons the hard way and through your own experiences. I have learned a lot from my experiences and thought to share some strategies that help my stress level as a manager. First, do not sweat the small stuff but stay firm with standards and expectations especially if they are reasonable and achievable. Second, be friendly, outgoing, compassionate, see both sides as a staff PT and center manager, and stick up for people that will stick up for you. Thirdly, if possible try to hire your own staff. New hires will not know anything else but your standards and expectations. It is much easier to start someone fresh then to change a staff that use to do it a certain way. Finally, try to relax and do not stress too much about the center manager role. Being a center manager should be fun, exciting, and also challenging. A good center manager is fun, firm, tough, a problem solver, and someone that your staff will stick up for and love working for. Your staff will not like everything that you say, do, or implement but if they like working for you and respect you then that is all you can ask for.

Chapter 31

Focus on Proper Form & Function

When treating any patient no matter what area of the body you are treating, it always comes back to what is causing the dysfunction, can we treat it in PT, and what is the normal function of that area. Most patients have pain and symptoms due to poor posture, muscular imbalances, muscular substitutions and structural dysfunctions. Unless the joint structure is impaired beyond repair and a structural defect is not a main cause of pain, symptoms, or functional limitation then physical therapy should help the patient.

Most therapists think that we get people better by making them do exercises correctly. Actually while that is important, people benefit the most from education about their condition, a proper patient specific home exercise program, and learning what will make them better outside of physical therapy. Patients are only in PT for about a month or two, which can amount to 6-12 visits. What the patients take with them and does on a daily or weekly basis outside of physical therapy is more important for long lasting benefit and results.

The easiest way to relate form and function for the human body is with general muscle action and functional muscle actions needed to perform every day actions such as walking, sitting, sit to stand, going up/down stairs, etc.. For example if you have a patient with a shoulder problem and the person cannot lift their arm to the side or behind their back then you have to think about the muscle action of the rotator cuff and anterior shoulder that may not be working correctly. They could be limited by ROM, joint mobility, and muscle strength but ultimately it is a deficit or dysfunction of their shoulder joint and/or rotator cuff muscles. You need to perform various special tests, examine their joint mobility, muscular flexibility, and the muscle actions/motions that perform the limited ROM and muscular contraction.

To maximize a patient's rehab potential, they need to show proper form, technique, and ROM while performing therapeutic exercises, flexibility, therapeutic activities, and neuromuscular re-education exercises. Proper exercise form and technique needs to be a major focus of all your treatments for all your patients due to the fact that most of your patients are suffering from muscular imbalances, poor posture, and functional muscle weaknesses. Most patient dysfunctions and symptoms can be corrected with proper posture, education of muscle function, and increasing muscle strength and flexibility. A lot of patients just want to come to PT, fly through their exercises and be out of their physical therapy treatment session as quickly as possible. To be a good PT you need to be a stickler and strict on exercise technique and form. Patients will usually show incorrect form due to muscular imbalances, compensation for weakness, and sometimes just pure laziness. As a medical professional you need to correct them and explain what they are doing wrong and why they should not be doing that.

With every patient, especially with patients who have had shoulder surgery, you need to break the compensation of tight, weak, and restricted muscles as soon as possible. If you do not then they will pick up bad habits like shoulder upper trap shrugging during shoulder elevation/flexion, forward head posture, and overworked rhomboids and scapular stabilizers. The shoulder is a very complex, mobile, and complicated joint and that is why you need work on proper shoulder kinematics, joint mobility, scapulohumeral rhythm, and ROM. If proper strength, flexibility, mobility, and scapulohumeral rhythm are not a major focus of treatment then they most likely will never regain full ROM, strength, flexibility, mobility, and proper shoulder kinematics which are necessary for all shoulder movements in all planes of motion.

We have all been to the gym and seen the guys who have improper unsafe lifting form. They lift barbells with every part of their bodies while doing bicep curls or quickly and unsafely strain when attempting to push or pull a lot of weight. Lifting improperly even with light weights can cause muscle strains, sprains, and traumatic arthritis. We work muscles and tendons in the gym and in PT while using good form and technique for safety and security of body and muscles. Education about proper lifting technique, form and posture is crucial for patient to maximize their rehab potential and to prevent future injuries. Most patients want to lift big weights and increase their strength but your patients might be in PT due to improper lifting, muscular imbalances, and altered shoulder kinematics. Lifting smaller weights with weakened muscles is what most people need in PT. Scapular depressor and retractors are typically weak in a lot of neck and shoulder patients. Thinking logically and developing a plan to improve muscular imbalances is what needs to be done for most patients. Remember you are only as strong as your weakest muscle, so normalizing muscular imbalances is vital.

Athletes and higher level patients are usually in PT for pain and dysfunction due to muscular imbalances. Baseball pitchers, soccer players, and volleyball players usually will have muscular imbalances where one muscle group is super strong and/or super tight based on the demands of the sports. Baseball players can usually develop shoulder internal and external rotation deficits. Soccer players may develop strong quads but have pretty weak hamstrings or gluteal muscles. When you focus on improving muscular balance, proper form, and increasing function you will improve patient outcomes and maximize your patients rehab potential.

Chapter 32

Athletes

For 2 months in 2009 I had the opportunity to do a student clinical rotation in the great outpatient orthopedic clinic of Champion Sports Medicine at St. Vincent's Hospital in Birmingham Alabama. Now for those who many not know, that clinic is very busy with high profile professional athletes under the care of the world famous Dr. James Andrews. Dr. Andrews is one of, if not the busiest orthopedic surgeon for shoulder, elbow, and knee orthopedic athletic injuries. He is mostly known for his surgeries with high profile athletes such as NFL quarterbacks, running backs, MLB pitchers, and NBA point guards among many others.

I learned a lot of the treatment principles, protocols, and exercises that I still use today and will use the rest of my physical therapy career. One of the biggest aspects of physical therapy I learned is that no matter who is injured or what the injury is, the patient care should not change. A professional athletes injury should not be more important that an amateur or non-athletes injury. Now, do not get me wrong a shoulder of a super bowl MVP quarterback is very important to the NFL, the team, and his fans but you do not treat it any differently (especially early on) than a person with the same exact injury or surgery that is not worth a couple million dollars. The only difference is the demand that the patient will be returning to and stressors that will be put back onto the injured area. The return to sport training, which starts around 3-4 month mark depending on the surgery, is the major difference of a high level professional athlete versus an amateur athlete.

Early treatment for all patients recovering from athletic injuries such as, a rotator cuff repair, ACL reconstruction, and meniscus repair is the same. The main focus in to gain functional

ROM as early as possible without stressing healing tissue. Most of the time, the early focus of PT deals with passive range of motion (PROM), active assistive range of motion (AAROM), isometric strength, proper posture, education, and decreasing inflammation.

Most people think that working with athletes is great and an amazing job, and for the most part it is. However, high profile athletes can be high maintenance, test your limits, and not accept what you are telling them about their condition and outcomes. Athletes hate missing time in their sports and want to be back playing as quickly as possible. They turn into workaholics, overachievers, and need to be watched very carefully. You give them a home exercise program (HEP) and they are doing it four times a day instead of twice a day like you said and doing twice the amount of repetitions it says for each exercise. Athletes are usually in better shape overall but healing time from an injury and after a surgery falls under certain categories and time frames. If an athlete breaks his leg, it will take 12 weeks to heal regardless if he wants it to heal faster or not. Most athletes hate to be injured and being out 12 weeks is unacceptable to most athletes. It is your job as a medical professional to do no harm and letting someone come back from injury too soon can cause a patient harm. In situations of conflict about a patient returning to sport, I feel that you have to tell them the truth about when they can return to their sport. Making them understand and educating them is usually the best way of resolving conflict about their injury.

Making an athlete feel that you are on their side and that you want them to play as quickly as they possibly can is what needs to be done for injured athletes. Athletes usually do not like bad news about injuries and only want to know when they will be able to return to their prior activity level. No matter what you tell athletes, they will want to come back sooner than what you say. If you tell them that they will be out for 3 weeks, they will say that they are coming back in 1-2 weeks. Athletes cannot accept being down with an injury but it is your job to make then accept it, even if they don't like it. I'd rather have an athlete rest another week or month so an injury can heal properly or recover from a surgery completely, so the athlete can play another 5 years or the rest of their lives at an amateur level.

There is nothing better than having a motivated patient that wants to get better and who will listen to their therapist. Athletes can be a lot of fun to treat and usually can perform fun higher level activities such as plyometrics, resisted backwards walking, monster walks, step downs, and more. Athletes can get injured for many different reasons but most injuries are commonly due to muscular imbalances, improper form, trauma, and repetitive stress. Improving function, posture, kinematics, mobility, correcting muscular imbalances, and increasing joint and muscle mobility should be a main focus for most patients. Athletes can injure themselves due to muscular imbalances and having restricted mobility besides suffering injury from trauma. Faulty kinematics and improper form must be corrected in order to maintain proper health and avoidance of injury or re-injury. For example if you see a patients knee going inward (genu valgum) during a squat, that must be corrected in order to prevent knee and hip pathologies from occurring or re-occurring.

A great piece of advice is to find out what demands are placed on the athlete from the sport/activity that they will be returning to. Everyone knows what football is but what are the demands of the position that your patient plays. How about if you have a gymnast who tore her ACL, do you know what muscles are activated during the phases of movement? What about the form and kinematics needed to properly perform that sport or activity? I had a gymnast and did not know exactly the demands of the activities that she would be returning to. Like everyone, I have seen gymnastics on television and could hypothesis what forces and muscles were used during each event. To get a better idea of what my patient would be returning to, I asked to see video and have them describe the motions, actions, and techniques that they would be doing in gymnastics. The patient's mom was a prior gymnast, so she could describe and even show some of the movements. I learned a lot about gymnastics and the demands of the leg muscles that were needed to properly perform the actions. YouTube is a great source of video for various things but for PT education you can see various sports injuries and what the demands of many sports are. There are tons of research articles that have studied the demands of certain sports and the muscle activation of certain exercises/activities. Staying educated and informed about muscle actions, activations, contractions, and injuries is a must for all patients but definitely for athletes. By knowing what the specific movement kinematics and muscle actions needed for most sports are, you can develop a successful plan of care to effectively treat your patients and return them to their prior level of function.

Chapter 33

Surgery and the Post-Surgical Patient

Thousands of surgeries are performed each year on thousands of different patients and body parts. Some of your best and worse patients will be recovering from post-surgery on some body party that they injured, hurt, or have worn down from years of abuse. I would love to say that every patient that received surgery for their ailments has gotten better and was back to their normal abilities after surgery. That is definitely not the case and is far from it. I see tons of patients who are actually worse after surgery then before when I saw them. Unless you have a major decline in function, strength, mobility, quality of life and/or it needs to be done to save your life, then surgery is not medically necessary and should be avoided. I would not rush to get surgery unless it was a last resort to fix my dysfunction, pain, symptoms, or ailments and that is what I tell all my patients.

A common statement made by most of my patients is that they do not want to have surgery or if they have already had surgery they do not want to have it again. The last thing I want for someone is for them to have surgery unless it is medically necessary for them to function properly with proper muscle function, mechanics, and safety. The last resort for any condition, injury, or dysfunction should be surgery. Unless someone is so debilitated or cannot function due to pain and symptoms surgery should not be done. Patients are very inclined to follow a PT program when there is an option of surgery if PT does not work to treat their condition. Patients for the most part do not want surgery and if PT will prevent them from having surgery then they will do it.

The good news is that most conditions can get better with PT without the need of surgery. The bad news is that for some conditions, no matter how much exercise you do, surgery has to be done. Major athletic injuries where something is torn, broken, or shattered will require surgery. For example for a torn ACL or femur fracture will require surgery to provide the necessary joint structure, stabilization, and repair of a physical defect. Following surgery, the MD will most likely send the patient for PT that the patient will attend for several weeks to months.

My favorite patients are post-surgical patients and mainly surgeries of the shoulder and knee. I like treating patients with various injuries, dysfunctions, pathologies, and symptoms but I must say that shoulders and knees are my favorite. Based on my experiences and education from clinical rotations and course work I feel that I know more about the pathologies and conditions of the shoulder and knee and how to treat them effectively. Also most shoulder and knee post-surgical patients are the most compliant with PT visits, exercises, and education as they need PT in order to return to their prior level of function, strength, and ability.

There have been several different protocols made by doctors and orthopedic surgeons. No matter what the protocol is or who made it, the main goal is to progressively work the patient in a controlled manner and to not over stress the healing tissue. Gaining functional ROM, isometric strength, patient education, proper posture, and decreasing pain and inflammation are the main goals. Following the simple healing times for post-surgical structures will make your life easier and provide a guideline for exercises. There is some debate to what truly healing time is but general guidelines that I follow are: 2-4 weeks the tissue is 50% healed, 6-8 weeks the tissue is 80% healed and at 12 weeks the tissue is 100% healed. Depending if the patient has co-morbidities like diabetes or performs activities that will decrease healing time such as smoking, then the patient may take longer to heal. When a tissue has healed then you can work it harder, stretcher it farther and place more stress on it.

When in doubt to how the patient is performing in PT or if you can progress the patient with higher level exercises, please contact the referring doctor. A team approach is usually best especially since the operating doctor will know more specifics of the involved structures that were operated on. All post-surgical patients will want to achieve the same goal of increasing their strength; ROM, mobility, stabilization, and function back to at least where they were before surgery. Most cases, especially with ACL patients, a patient will actually be stronger in the surgical leg/limb than the non-injured/repaired side when their rehab is complete.

A home exercise program (HEP) is important for all patients but extremely important for the post-surgical patients that you will be treating. The last thing you want is for your patients to be positioning themselves wrong, having poor posture, not using the appropriate modalities, and poor or improper compliance with the exercises that you give them. If a patient is not compliant with the HEP you give them on the first or second treatment, it is usually pretty obvious. The patient will have more pain, less mobility, and more difficulty then the last time you saw them. Communication of what is expected with compliance of their HEP and what may happen if they do not abide by your program is necessary in assuring compliance. For example, if a patient does not position their leg properly after an ACL repair then they might never get full extension. Full extension is necessary for walking, playing sports, and general getting around. Gaining full extension is easy if the patient performs basic positioning and exercises at home but only if they actually do it. If the patient does not follow the HEP, then the surgeon may have to remove scar tissue by having another surgery and the patient definitely does not want that.

Constant communication about the patients rehab, progress, and future level of PT and exercises is crucial. People get bored in PT and someone recovering from surgery is already pretty weak and debilitated. The last thing a post-surgical patient wants to do is to come to PT and do basic exercises and feel that they are not really working their muscles. People want to feel challenged and that they are constantly making progress and being done with PT. By adding a couple new exercises and letting the patient know that they are doing well and we can progress the exercises next visit or pretty soon, the patients will feel that they are making progress and moving in the right direction.

Most post-surgical patients hate that they had to have surgery and want to recover quickly. When a patient is too motivated to get better, you have to worry about over stressing healing tissue. If a patient re-injures their repaired tissue then the doctor will be extremely unhappy, the patient will need more surgery, and the PT office will look bad. None of those options are good and need to be avoided. Working too hard too fast is never good and needs to be avoided. No matter what you do before the 12 week mark after surgery the healing tissue is not fully healed. Twelve weeks is what needs to be common knowledge to therapists and their patients, as that time frame needs to be achieved before you can start higher level activities. Patients will ask all the time, "When can I do this or when can I do that?" I usually reply after 3 months from your surgery date we will perform tests to try higher level activities. Twelve weeks is the earliest to try higher demand activities and needs to be constantly told to some patients.

Remember, not all patients will be the same even if they had the same surgery. Not all rotator cuff patients or ACL patients are the same. People will be of different ages, activities levels, and prior levels of function. Some may heal faster or slower but the main focus is the gain functional ROM, strength, mobility, and stabilization without over stressing healing tissue. Think about what tissue was repaired, and be careful with exercises that may work that tissue. Passive ROM (PROM) can be done right way as long as the patient is not fighting the movement or muscle guarding. After a patient has reached certain milestones of healed tissue, try a simple screen of ROM and strength before progressing with higher level activities. If all else fails or that you are unsure about what a patient can or cannot do, call and communicate with the doctor and his staff. Communication with the doctor and patient is extremely important and can only improve your patient outcomes and progress towards your PT goals.

Chapter 34

Manual Therapy Does Not Equal Massage Therapy

Being a certified manual therapist, I have a little bias to the benefit of performing manual therapy. I am not alone as the research shows great efficacy of performing manual therapy along with therapeutic exercise. That being said, manual therapy does not equal massage therapy. Manual therapy and massage therapy are two different avenues that share similar techniques but manual therapy consists of much more education, research, and techniques. Manual therapy is a great tool that needs to be used by all therapists on almost every patient in some form or fashion. A therapist needs to get a hands on with a patient for ROM, stretching, joint mobility, flexibility, soft tissue mobilization, and PNF patterns.

There is nothing wrong with massage therapy but I do not want my 7 year doctorate of physical therapy considered equal to a couple month long certification of massage therapy. I am not trying to put down massage therapy as a profession but I must make this statement about PT and massage therapy. A lot of doctors send their patient to us for hot pack, ultrasound, and massage. Those patients usually do not like coming to see us, because you will be doing stretching, strengthening exercises, some soft tissue mobilizations, maybe some ROM, education, and a home exercise program (HEP) with stretching, strengthening, and flexibility on it. Massage therapy is not covered under insurance plans and doctors send their patients to us expecting us to give palliative care treatments and massage.

Once you have been practicing PT for a couple years, you will see a lot of interesting things from doctors and prescriptions for PT. I cannot count how many times I have seen PT prescriptions or have taken phone calls about PT treatments with massage, ultrasound, hot packs, and basic palliative care spa type treatments. I want no part of a clinic that takes patients in for that. I know some PT clinics that do that type of palliative spa type treatment for every patient that comes in. I believe PT should be a mix of manual therapy, therapeutic exercise, patient education, and HEP. Having patients come in for massage will not truly get them better in the long run, it will hurt the therapists hands, shoulders, and backs, and not help anyone if we only do that spa type palliative care.

If massage therapy was ordered for a patient, the MD will send them to physical therapy due to the fact that massage therapy is not covered by most insurance companies. So doctors knowing that, send them to physical therapy wanting massage for their patients. Doctors tell patients that I will send you to PT for massage and paint a picture of massage and palliative care. That is a major problem that I have seen with doctors referring for massage or modalities only. A patient will not get better, stronger, and improve functional impairment with massage, hot packs, ultrasound, and electrical stimulation only. When a patient calls our office inquiring about massage, I make sure that my front desk person knows to reply with, "Yes, we do soft tissue techniques like massage but you will be doing exercises and not just getting a massage for an hour."

Massage will not be reimbursed if it is billed under the massage CPT code. If massage techniques are performed than they must be billed under the manual therapy CPT code. Massage is not classified as medically necessary and will never be reimbursed by insurances. Manual therapy is skilled therapeutic intervention and will be reimbursed on the manual therapy CPT code. It might seem confusing or knit-picking but that is how insurances work and you need to know to play the game to maximize your revenue.

Chapter 35

Make It Fun

     No matter what you are doing; it is always better if you can make it fun. Physical therapy should be fun and a joy for patients to go to. If your patient is not having fun, then they are less likely to come back for future visits. Patients get bored just like anyone else, so you have to make it fun and change it up when you can. When possible, at the end of a treatment, tell the patient that you will be adding something next visit and stepping up their exercises. The patient will leave thinking that they are getting better, making progress towards PT goals, and getting some new exercises to help further there treatment and ultimate goal of returning to their prior level of function.

     I know myself if I am bored with something or activity then I will move onto to something else that holds my interest or is more exciting. PT should be fun and exciting when possible. Now if someone is a couple weeks post-surgery then you will be limited by the activities and exercises that you can perform based on healing time and limitations of the surgery. When someone is there for general aches and pains, arthritis, or at a higher level of treatment following 3 to 4 months post-surgery then you can mix up the exercises or add something fun that the patient will look forward to doing every treatment. Even if the patient is there for another body part, adding some fun activity that may not work the injured area is ok. If the patient enjoys doing the activity and is fun and safe for the patient to perform then try it out. Making your patients happy along with getting them better is good for business and your general well-being at work.

     Knowing the muscle action, joint kinematics, muscle function and how that motion is related to your patient's condition should be a good reason why to have a patient perform an exercise. For example, the hamstrings of the leg perform knee flexion and hip extension. You can work the hamstrings by a variety of exercises as long as that exercise performs knee flexion. So for the patient that has some leg weakness, post knee surgery, and/or muscular imbalances performing knee flexion and hamstring strengthening, stretching, and flexibility is a must. That being said, you have some freedom as a therapist on how to contract those muscles and what exercises to have the hamstring work efficiently. So mix it up, don't be afraid to think outside the box with exercises as long as you and the patient can safely perform the exercises with good form and technique.

Another overlooked way to make it fun is the music or television station you have on in the clinic. In our clinic, we have a radio that plays a mix of music from the 70s to the 90s that is mostly rock n roll. The majority of PT patients will have grown up with or lived in the era of the 70s and 80s and will enjoy listening that music. Knowing your crowd and patient population is important for how to make them happy and enjoy the environment of the clinic. Fun exciting music is pretty important to the vibe and feel of the clinic. If you don't have music in your clinic then you should try it out and you will see how it changes the atmosphere and mood of your staff, patients, and clinic.

Chapter 36

A Team of Two

   I like to have the motto of "A team of two", which means that the therapist and patient will work as a team to improve the patients function, decrease their pain and symptoms, and return the patient to their prior level of function if possible. For any patient to truly maximize their rehab potential, they need to be compliant with a home exercise program (HEP) and the education that they receive from their PT. Patients are usually only in therapy for a maximum of 3 hours a week for about 3-4 months, which is not a long time at all considering that we have 24 hours in a day and 7 days a week. They need to be compliant with what you give them to do and listen to what not to do at home. Some of the best treatment for patients is basic information and education of their condition and how to get them better. If you can teach someone how to get better then they usually are more reliable and compliant with their HEP. If someone knows and understands why they are doing something or why not to do something, they will be more inclined to follow and/or "buy in" to the treatment plan of care.

   People like to know that you are trying to get them better and that you are giving them the power to make it happen. By working together as a team of two, you can work together to improve their function and reach their goals. Anyone who has played sports likes the feeling of being part of a team and surrounded by people that share the same views and goals as you. In sports, the goal is usually to win a championship; in PT that goal is usually to come back from an injury, dysfunction, and/or pathology better and stronger than before.

   Whether you like it or not, you and the patient are a team. You work together in the clinic and the patient follows through with a home program and education that you teach them. The patient will maximize their rehab potential if they show good compliance with their HEP and the therapist keeps improving and increasing the activities and exercises that the patient can perform in PT. When the patient can successfully perform exercises with minimal/ no difficulty and pain or symptoms then it is the job of the therapist to increase the demand of the exercises either by adding new exercises, increasing sets and or reps, or using a new piece of equipment. As a team working together like a coach and a player, the patient can usually reach a higher level of function, strength, and ability while in PT. "A team of two" will always beat a single person. As a patient and therapist working together, the sky is the limit of how far a patient can achieve with their dysfunction, impairment, and rehab.

Chapter 37

Home Exercise Program

 A home exercise program (HEP) is necessary for most patients that come to PT. A patient specific home program needs to be given to patients so they can maximize their rehab potential and work on exercises at home. A patient is only in PT for a couple hours a week for a couple weeks. A couple hours a week is not a long enough time for a patient to truly get better and focus on the factors that may have caused their pain, symptoms, and dysfunction in the first place.

 When most people think of home exercise programs, they think of exercises with bands or weights. A home exercise program should consist of anything and everything that a patient can safely perform at home and will benefit from doing. I like to provide exercises that focus on improving a patient's flexibility, mobility, range of motion, and strength along with self-care and education. Making a note on an exercise sheet about proper posture, using ice or heat, and resting positions after a surgery are very important. A written home exercise sheet needs to be given to each patient as they can refer to the sheet when they forgot what you told them to do. The sheet needs to be explained very well and reviewed with the patient. Reviewing the exercise sheet and answering any and all patient questions will limit compliance issues and problems.

 During the initial evaluation, or at latest the patients' second visit, I provide them with a written home exercise sheet. The home exercise program needs to be specific to the patient and will cover areas of need that the patient can safely perform. I stress that aspect of safety, as the last thing you want to do is to have a patient get hurt with exercises that you told them to do. For example, a balance patient may want a home exercise program but for safety reasons you may not be able to give them much of a program. Vestibular and balance training needs to be treated with the care and supervision of a trained professional along with a carefully designed home program. To increase a patient's balance, you must work on balance activities, increase leg strength, and improve the vestibular system. That can only be done with a skilled professional and most people do not have one of those at home, so higher level static and dynamic balance activities should be avoided in a home program. Balance activities, such as having a patient with their eyes open or closed standing on one leg or an unstable surface will require a patient to be supervised and guarded by a PT. For vestibular and balance patients, I try to make a program that will stress the vestibular system in a controlled manner. For example, I will have the patient perform exercises while seated and at no risk of falling. While seated I will have them look at targets with their eyes only and having their head remain still or have their eyes remain fixed on a target and have their head move either up and down or side to side. They still are stressing their vestibular system but by having them seated instead of standing, there is minimal danger of falling and injuring themselves.

Home exercise programs are best designed for the treatment of orthopedic injuries, muscular imbalances, and post – surgical patients. The exercises need to be chosen based on the benefit to the patient, patient compliance, and safety. Exercise band (e.g. thera-band) exercises are great if a patient has them at home or plans on buying them. At our clinic we sell bands, so the patient can learn some exercises with bands and pick up a green or blue resistance band to continue the exercises at home. If a patient had surgery then the HEP will usually consist of exercises to improve ROM and strength of the tissues that were repaired but in a safe manner as to never overstress healing tissue. For example, a patient had rotator cuff surgery and we are seeing the patient 2 weeks after surgery. You want to give them a specific HEP to work on increasing ROM and scapular stabilization recruitment. I would give them some passive and active assisted ROM that can be done with a cane, umbrella, or broom, I would give them some scapular retractor exercises, pendulums to work on passive ROM, and some table slides to help improve shoulder flexion ROM. The exercises can be done with minimal or even no equipment and they would be relevant to the patient since we want to safely improve the patients ROM and scapular position following shoulder surgery.

A written home exercise program can be made through various computer programs, pre-made print outs, and making copies of exercises from sheets or exercise cards. If you see a lot of patients will similar diagnosis, conditions, or surgeries, than you might want to design pre-made sheets that can be used for several patients. I like to use a combination of pre-made sheets and exercises cards that I can copy and edit to make a specific HEP for my patients. I make one copy for the patient and another copy for their chart. I cannot count how many times I have had patients ask me for another copy of their exercises and I can easily make a copy of the sheet that I put in their chart. A chart copy is a good way to show that you have documented proof of providing a written HEP for the patient and also have a reference of their first HEP when you want to advance their program.

Home exercise programs should be designed as being two levels, one as a beginner level and the next as an advanced level. When possible, try to give a basic program for post-surgical and deconditioned patients and an advanced program for higher level athletes and when a patient is ready to move past the basic PT program. A patient needs to show proper form and techniques in the clinic before you can trust that they will perform the activities correctly at home. Be sure to educate and the review with the patient the proper number of sets, reps, and how many times a day a patient should complete the program. Patients need to show proper compliance with PT visits and exercises along with home exercise programs to achieve good rehab potential. Poor compliance can be if a patient does not do the program at all or they do it too much. Athletes and highly motivated patients may do twice as many exercises, sets, and reps as you tell them, thinking that it will get them to heal faster and finish with PT quicker. Patient compliance with all aspects of PT needs to be established early and often. The last thing you want is for a patient to do twice as many sets and reps and potentially hurt themselves by causing a muscle strain or another injury. I have not seen a patient hurt themselves with performing a HEP, but some have come close.

Education is a major part of PT and needs to be a major part of patient home exercise programs. Teaching someone what to do and more importantly what not do, needs to be a standard for all therapists. I am a firm believer that you cannot educate or teach someone too much information. That mindset is a great principle regarding a patient's diagnosis, condition, and HEP as teaching a patient about their condition and will help them get better. When I educate someone about heat or ice, I make a note to write that information down on their HEP sheet. Most of the time, I have to hand write information on a sheet that contains exercises, but I want to make sure that the patient has written instructions on specific care while at home. If I only tell someone what to do, they are most likely to forget what I told them completely or partially. A home exercise program is a cheat sheet for exercises and information. If something is important for a patient to remember or to do at home, than it is important to take the extra couple of minutes to write it down so they will understand. Providing quality care and information in the PT clinic and with a HEP is what PT is all about. Please do not underestimate the power of your information and education in the clinic and with home exercise programs.

Chapter 38

Modalities

    Modalities, for those who may not know, are what we commonly call heat, ice, electrical stimulation, and ultrasound. They usually play a small role in my day to day care for patients. Of course I use hot packs, cold packs, electrical stimulation, and occasionally ultrasound but I definitely do not rely on them for the main part of my daily treatments. If a person needs modalities more than any part of skilled physical therapy treatment, then I will usually discharge to a home program where they can do that at home. We commonly educate patients on the use of home electrical stimulation units that they or their insurance has purchased. Electrical stimulation and mainly a Trans-Electrical-Neuromuscular-Stimulation or TENS current is most commonly used for treatment in the clinic to manage and minimize/eliminate pain.

    The best ways I think about the use of modalities is to use common sense and not to waste your time with something that has been shown in research article to have limited results. For example, therapeutic ultrasound is the biggest culprit of a modality that has not been shown to help many dysfunctions/injuries in PT. So therefore I do not perform it on a regular basis. I mainly use hot packs, cold packs, electrical stimulation, and iontophoresis. I use heat for arthritic patients or to loosen up tight, tender, and restricted muscles and ice to decrease inflammation and swelling. Now with all that being said, you might have to use heat on patient that you normally would use ice for and vice versa based on patient preference/request. Unless using a certain modality is contraindicated for that patient, then I see no problem putting ice on a patient that I might normally use heat on. Remember the customer is always right, and the use of a modality is a good example of how to listen to your patients and make them feel that they are listened to and you are honoring their requests.

When used appropriately, cold packs, hot packs, and electrical stimulation can provide relief from pain, symptoms, swelling, and general aches and pains. Most of the time we use a hot pack or cold back along with the use electrical stimulation (TENS current), so you can get a better bang for your buck and relief from symptoms. If a patient is in moderate to severe pain, I will generally perform some soft tissue mobilization and stretching followed by the hot or cold pack and electrical stimulation due to the fact that they are in distress and you need to calm that down before you can move on with further advanced exercises and/or treatment.

Modalities are a great tool to add to your PT session treatments and patient care. I do not and will never recommend modality only care. Some doctors and patients will only want modalities but I try to add some exercises, education and treatment along with the modalities. Modalities alone have not been shown to provide anything but temporary pain relief. For some patients, that temporary pain relief is all that they want from PT. Most patients want to improve their function, strength, stabilization, posture, range of motion, and flexibility which cannot be achieved from modalities alone.

You can and should make your own decisions about modalities but the use of modalities should be determined based on will it make the patient better or not. I do not like to waste my time with pointless modalities and treatments, so I treat patients with evidence based medicine, techniques, and modalities. No research article or study has ever shown that the use of modalities alone to have cured or provided enough long term symptom relief and improved function. You be the judge to how you use modalities but please make your decisions based on clinically relevant research, articles, and common sense.

Chapter 39

Simple PT Principles for Proper Patient Care

1) Keep your muscles Loose, Strong, and Flexible

2) Create a healing environment

3) Eccentric Muscle Contractions Are Great for Tendonitis and Functional Strengthening

4) Mobilize Hypomobilities, Stabilize Hypermobilities

5) If it is not obvious, then it probably is not a big concern or cannot be treated in PT

6) When In doubt, treat impairments, imbalances, posture, and weaknesses

7) Team of Two, need to stress the importance of PT, compliance with HEP & patient education

8) Do No Harm

9) The Costumer/Patient is always right...To an Extent

10) Re-schedule patients instead of canceling their appointment

11) Do Not Over Stress Healing Tissue

12) Do Not Have Patients Waiting Even If They Are Early

13) Post-Surgery at 2-4 weeks = 50% healed, 6-8 weeks = 80% healed, 12 weeks = 100% healed

14) People like to be challenged and progressed in PT, do not keep the patient performing the same boring exercises

15) Treat others how you would want to be treated

16) Function, Function, Function Need to improve function for all patients

17) Nobody cares about your problems; the patients are there to get better

18) You can never explain and teach too much about their condition

19) Document properly, safety first & always, and have fellow staff witness patient care when possible

20) Do not underestimate the power of what you are telling people

21) Be truthful when appropriate even if the patient will not like the truths that are telling them
22) Patients sometimes lie about their condition & you need to observe body language, facial expressions & signs
23) All patient are not created equal
24) You are only as strong as your weakest muscle
25) Some patients will not listen to you while others will listen to everything that you say
26) Make it fun, everyone likes to have fun
27) Must be able to adapt and change treatment intervention according to patient response, body language, & other signs
28) Patient trust must be earned and kept during all patient interactions
29) Contact with referring physicians is a must to provide quality care for all patients
30) A great PT will maintain interest with all their patients
31) 30 minutes of treatment is better than not seeing a patient
32) Make patients feel that you are going the extra mile for them
33) Do not let a patient sit in the waiting room for more than 5 -10 minutes
34) Document properly so there is no loss of care when another therapist treats your patients
35) Find the good in every situation and with every patient

These simple principles are great guidelines to help you treat patients. If you can perform several of these principles with all of your patients then you will be very successful and provide high quality PT in your clinic. Some of these principles are easy to say but hard to do. Just like most things in life, the more experience and knowledge you obtain the better you will be at something. These are not intended to be anything more than a simple guide to patient care.

Chapter 40

7 Most Common Musculoskeletal Injured Areas & Pathologies
<u>Neck</u>: Disc, Stenosis, OA, Facet, Whiplash, DJD, Instability
<u>Shoulders:</u> RTC, Biceps, Labrum, AC, Impingement, Bursitis, Frozen Shoulder, Dislocation, Humeral Fx, Tendonitis, Strain, Sprain
<u>Elbow/Forearm</u>: Tennis Elbow, Golfers Elbow, UCL, Elbow Dislocation
<u>Low Back</u>: Disc, Stenosis, Facet, SI, Instability, Strain, Spondylolisthesis, Sciatica, Piriformis Syndrome
<u>Hips</u>: Labrum, Bursitis, OA, Tight Hip Flexors, Tight IT Band, Glut Medius Weakness, Femur Fx, THR
<u>Knees</u>: Ligaments, Meniscus, Patella Tendon, OA, Sprain, Jumper's Knee, Chondromalacia Patella, TKR
<u>Ankles/Foot:</u> Stress Fx, Ankle Fx, Sprain, Achilles Tendon, Plantar Fascia

Low Back, Neck, Shoulder, and Knee pathologies are the most common treated areas seen in outpatient PT. Low back pain is the most common complaint in PT and the 2nd reason why people go to the doctor each year. The 1st reason is the common cold or flu. Taking care of your back is vital to prolonged health and should be a focus of general wellness. Neck pain & pathologies are another common reason why people seek treatment in PT. Neck pain is very treatable with patient education, changing seated and standing postures, and strengthening of the smaller muscles of the neck.

Shoulders and knee pathologies are common due to traumatic injuries of sports, general wear and tear, and muscular imbalances. Compliance with a home exercise program of stretching, strengthening and stabilization exercises can usually improve pain and symptoms that most patients are having. As with anything in the human body some conditions and pathologies will require a doctor's care and possible surgical intervention. Please consult your doctor first before starting PT.

Chapter 41

Fun Facts

There are 227 PT schools in the U.S. and 1 in Puerto Rico

The biggest muscle in the body is the gluteus maximus muscle.

You have all the muscle fiber you will ever have at birth.

The human tongue consists of sixteen separate muscles.

Your hands may not be the biggest part of your body, but they have 20 muscles

The sartorius muscle is the longest muscle in the body. This muscle runs from the hip area diagonally across the thigh to the inside of the knee.

Of the 206 bones in the skeletal system, 52 of them make up both of the feet. Injuries to the foot can be debilitating.

Humans & giraffes have the same number of cervical vertebrae; giraffe vertebrae are just much longer.

The hand has 27 bones, 8 of which are in the wrist. Hand injuries account for nearly 10% of hospital emergency department visits

PT Tips

Did you know that the biggest muscle in the body is the Gluteus Maximus?

The Gluteus Maximus does External Rotation and Extension of the Hip joint, supports the Extended Knee through the iliotibial tract, and is a chief antigravity muscle in sitting and Abduction of the hip. Besides attracting the opposite sex, it also provides stability for the low back and needs to be kept strong for activities such as sprinting, squatting, cutting, and jumping. To work the Gluteus Maximus you need to perform squats, lunges, hip extensions, hamstring curls, and gluteal isometric squeezes. A weak Gluteus Maximus has been linked to Knee, Foot and Back Pain.

PT Tips

Ice vs. Heat

Ice is used as an anti-inflammatory and should be used to reduce swelling and for an acute injury (1-7 days).Heat is good for muscle aches and joint pain and is mainly used for sore muscles and arthritis. You do not have to alternate between them to help flush the area, just stick with one of the two. If you are going to use either of them only keep them on for about 20 minutes at a time and check the skin after you are done to make there is no irritation, burns, blisters, or skin breakdown.

PT Tips

Sciatica: The term Sciatica is used to describe a symptom rather than a specific disease. Some use it to mean any pain starting in the lower back and going down the leg. Others use the term more specifically to mean a nerve dysfunction caused by compression of one or more lumbar or sacral nerve roots from a spinal disc herniation.

Sciatica can be caused by a variety of reasons but is mainly due to compression of a peripheral nerve in the lumbar spine or pelvis by the Piriformis muscle. Sciatica can be treated in a variety of ways but is mainly treated by stretching, strengthening, and tissue mobilization. The Piriformis is an External Rotator of the Hip and needs to be stretched by performing Internal Rotation of the Hip by either lying down on you back or seated.

PT Tips

Did you know that the Rotator Cuff is actually 4 muscles and Rotator Cuff problems are usually due to 4 common causes? Common causes of Rotator Cuff injuries include:

Normal wear and tear. Increasingly after age 40, normal wear and tear on your rotator cuff can cause a breakdown of collagen in the cuff's tendons and muscles. This makes them more prone to degeneration and injury. With age, you may also develop calcium deposits within the cuff or arthritic bone spurs that can pinch or irritate your rotator cuff.

Poor posture. When you slouch your neck and shoulders forward, the space where the rotator cuff muscles reside can become smaller. This can allow a muscle or tendon to become pinched under your shoulder bones (including your collarbone), especially during overhead activities, such as throwing.

Falling. Using your arm to break a fall or falling on your arm can bruise or tear a rotator cuff tendon or muscle.

Lifting or pulling. Lifting an object that's too heavy or doing so improperly especially overhead can strain or tear your tendons or muscles. Likewise, pulling something, such as a high-poundage archery bow, may cause an injury.

Repetitive stress. Repetitive overhead movement of your arms can stress your rotator cuff muscles and tendons, causing inflammation and eventually tearing. This occurs often in athletes, especially baseball pitchers, swimmers and tennis players.

PT Tips

Our muscles often work in pairs so that they can pull in different or opposite directions.

A common cause of shoulder, mid back, and neck pain is due to muscle imbalances, poor posture, and improper lifting form. You need to be well rounded and work on all your muscles. Beach muscles (Chest, Biceps, & Shoulders) need to take a back seat if you are experiencing shoulder, neck, and or mid back pain at rest and while working out. Muscle pain and symptoms can be easily corrected with proper posture, more pulling and less pressing strength, and using correct form.

The Bench press, Military Press, and Lat Pull downs are great muscle builders but are very common exercises that can cause pain, strain, and structural problems such as bone spurs in shoulders, rotator cuff dysfunction, and shoulder impingement. Heavy weight while doing pressing exercises should be avoided for most people unless correct form and technique can be maintained while lifting heavy weight.

Appendix

Manual Muscle Testing (MMT) Grades

0 = None   No visible or palpable contraction

1 = Trace   **Visible or palpable contraction (No ROM)**

2- = Poor -   Partial ROM, gravity eliminated

2 = Poor   **Full ROM, gravity eliminated**

2+ = Poor +   Gravity eliminated/slight resistance or < 1/2 range against gravity

3- = Fair -   > 1/2 but < Full ROM, against gravity

3 = Fair   **Full ROM against gravity**

3+ = Fair +   Full ROM against gravity, slight resistance

4- = Good -   Full ROM against gravity, mild resistance

4 = Good   **Full ROM against gravity, moderate resistance**

4+ = Good +   Full ROM against gravity, almost full resistance

5 = Normal   **Max Resistance**

Special Tests

UE
Speeds Test, Full Can, Apley's Scratch Test, Gerber Lift Off, Drop Arm, Belly Press, Neer Impingement, Active O'Brien Test, AC Joint Compression

LE
Lachman's, Poster Sag, Valgus and Varus Tests, active SLR, McConnell Chondromalacia, Apley's Compression, McMurray Test, Thomas Test, Ober's Test, Noble's Compression, Talar Tilt, Kleiger

Spine
Straight Leg Raise, Active Straight Leg Raise, FABER, Traction, Upper Limb Tension Test 1-4, Vertebral Artery Test, Slump, Shoulder ABD Test, Foraminal Compression

There are hundreds of special tests for the human body. The lists of tests (p.120) are tests that we perform on our patients and have been found to be effective and show good sensitivity and/or specificity. The listed tests are not intended to be the only special tests that should performed on your patients but merely to provide some guidance and help when evaluating patients.

Deep Tendon Reflexes (DTR)	DTR Grading Scale
C5 = Biceps	0 = Absent
C6 = Brachioradialis	1+ = Diminished/Sluggish
C7 = Triceps	2+ = Normal
L4 = Quad	3+ = Brisk
S1 = Achilles Tendon	4+ = Pathological/Clonus

Palpation

Use your middle finger as it has been found to be more sensitive to discriminate between tight, sensitive, and tender tissue.

Common anatomical structures for palpation and areas that you should try to palpate/examine during your evaluation:

UE

Biceps , Supraspinatus, Infraspinatus, Forearm Flexors & Extensors, Pec Major & Minor, Upper Trap, Triceps, Subscapularis, Deltoids

LE

Quads, Hamstrings, IT Band, Gluteal Muscles, Gastrocnemius, Soleus, Achilles Tendon, Patella Tendon, Quad Tendon, Iliopsoas, Adductors, Knee Joint Lines, Medial & Lateral Ankles

Spine

Suboccipitals, Rhomboids, QL, Erector Spinae, Lower Trap, Latissimus Dorsi, PSIS, ASIS, Scalenes, Levator Scapulae, SCM

Common Joint Mobility Glides

Shoulder & Hip Joint

Flexion: Posterior & Inferior   **Extension:** Anterior

Abduction: Anterior & Inferior   **External Rotation:** Anterior

Internal Rotation: Posterior

Elbow

Flexion: Anterior   **Extension:** Posterior

Supination: Anterior   **Pronation:** Posterior

Wrist

Flexion: Posterior   **Extension:** Anterior

Knee

Flexion: Posterior   **Extension:** Anterior

Ankle

Dorsiflexion: Posterior   **Plantar Flexion:** Anterior

Commonly Used ICD-9 Codes

Upper Extremity

726.0 Adhesive Capsulitis   **726.10 Rotator Cuff Tear/Sprain**

726.12 Biceps Tendonitis   **726.19 Shoulder Impingement**

813.41 Colle's Fx   **840.7 SLAP Tear**

Lower Extremity

715.16 Osteoarthritis of the Knee   **V43.65 Total Knee Replacement**

732.4 Osgood Schlatter's Disease

715.95 Osteoarthritis of the Hip   **V43.64 Total Hip Replacement**

836.1 Meniscus tear lateral   **836.2 Meniscus tear medial**

Spine

722.10 Sciatica   **724.2 Lumbago**

723.1 Cervicalgia   **847.0 Cervical Strain**

722.10 Herniated Disc   **723.4 Cervical Radiculitis**

353.0 Brachial Plexus Lesion   **724.1 Pain Thoracic Spine**

Medicare ICD-9 Codes

723.1 Neck Pain/Cervicalgia

724.1 Pain In Thoracic Spine

724.2 Low Back Pain/Lumbago

724.5 Backache

727.81 Contracture of Tendon

729.5 Pain In Limb

719.7 Difficulty Walking

781.2 Abnormality of Gait

719.41 Joint Pain Shoulder

719.42 Joint Pain Upper Arm

719.43 Joint Pain Forearm

719.44 Joint Pain Hand

719.45 Joint Pain Pelvis

719.46 Joint Pain Lower Leg

719.47 Joint Pain Ankle

719.49 Joint Pain Multiple Jts

Medicare Units

8-22 Minutes = 1

38-52 Minutes = 3

68-82 Minutes = 5

23-37 Minutes = 2

53-67 Minutes = 4

Medicare units are calculated from time based treatment codes only, such as Therapeutic Exercise, Manual Therapy, Neuromuscular Re-Education, and Therapeutic Activities. Ice, Hot Packs, Electrical Stimulation, Ultrasound, Traction, and other modalities do NOT count towards Medicare treatment unit time.

CPT Codes

97001: PT Initial Evaluation

97002: PT Re-Evaluation

97110: Therapeutic Exercise

97112: Neuromuscular Re-Education

97116: Gait Training

97140: Manual Therapy

97530: Therapeutic Activities

97535: Self-Care/Home Management

Dermatomes & Myotomes

Dermatomes

C4	Upper Trap
C5	Lateral deltoid area/Lateral arm
C6	Lateral forearm & thumb/Index finger
C7	Posterior arm/forearm into digit 3
C8	Ulnar border of hand into digit 5, Distal ½ of medial forearm
T1	Medial arm & proximal ½ of forearm
L2	Upper anterior thigh to mid medial thigh
L3	Front of thigh to medial aspect of knee
L4	Front of thigh anterior to knee, down medial leg
L5	Lateral leg to dorsum of foot & web space (1-2)
S1	Lateral foot & calf region
S2	Posterior thigh

Myotomes

C4	Shoulder Elevation
C5	Shoulder Abduction, Elbow Flexion, External Rotation
C6	Elbow Flexion, Supination, Wrist Extension
C7	Elbow Extension, Wrist Flexion, Finger Extension
C8	Thumb Extension, Finger Flexion, Ulnar Deviation
T1	Digit 5 Abduction or Abduction/Adduction of digits 2-5
L2	Hip Flexion, Hip Adduction
L3	Knee Extension
L4	Ankle Dorsiflexion
L5	Great Toe Extension
S1	Ankle Eversion, Ankle Plantar Flexion
S2	Ankle Plantar Flexion, Knee Flexion

There is great variance between sources of specific dermatome and myotome innervation. The above list is merely a summary from one source. Please consult other texts for more information.

Range Of Motion (ROM)

Hip
Flexion 0 – 120
Extension 0-30
Hyperextension -10
ABD 0 – 50
ADD 0 - 30
ER 0 – 45
IR 0 – 45

Shoulder
Flexion 0 – 180
Extension 0 – 50
ABD 0 – 180
ADD 50-75
Hor ABD 0 – 45
Hor ADD 0 – 130
ER & IR 0 – 100

PIP
Flexion 0 - 120
Extension 0

DIP
Flexion 0 – 80
Extension 0

Knee
Flexion 0 – 135
Extension 0 – (-10)

Elbow
Flexion 0 – 150
Extension 0 – (-10)
Pronation 0 – 90
Supination 0 – 90

Thumb MCP
Flexion 0 - 70
Extension 0
ABD 0 - 50

Ankle
PF 0- 50
DF 0 -20

Wrist
Flexion 0 – 80
Extension 0 - 70
Radial Deviation 0 - 20
Ulnar Deviation 0 -30

Thumb IP
Flexion 0 - 80
Extension 0

Foot
Inversion 0 - 35
Eversion 0 - 25

MTP joints
Flexion 0 - 30
Extension 0 – (-10)
ABD 0 - 25

MCP joints
Flexion 0 - 90
Extension 0 - 30

IP joints of toes
Flexion 0 - 50
Extension 0 – (-5)

Normative Values for ROM will greatly vary for each individual. A good predictor of normal ROM for a patient is to compare the non-involved side if the non-involved side had no prior injury, surgery, or problems. The ROM values listed above are a good basis for how much ROM a patient should have and will need to perform functional tasks and activities of daily living.

www.ingramcontent.com/pod-product-compliance
Lightning Source LLC
Chambersburg PA
CBHW051807170526
45167CB00005B/1915